Hypertension

Hypertension
COMMUNITY CONTROL OF HIGH BLOOD PRESSURE

Julian Tudor Hart MB, BChir, DCH, FRCP, FRCGP

General Practitioner,
Glyncorrwg Health Centre, West Glamorgan

FOREWORD TO THE FIRST EDITION BY THE LATE

Sir George Pickering FRS, MD, FRCP

Regius Professor of Medicine
University of Oxford

SECOND EDITION

CHURCHILL LIVINGSTONE
EDINBURGH LONDON MELBOURNE AND NEW YORK 1987

CHURCHILL LIVINGSTONE
Medical Division of Longman Group UK Limited

Distributed in the United States of America by
Churchill Livingstone Inc., 1560 Broadway, New
York, N. Y. 10036, and by associated companies,
branches and representatives throughout the world.

First edition 1980
Second edition 1987

ISBN 0-443-03152-5

British Library Cataloguing in Publication Data
Hart, Julian Tudor
  Hypertension: community control of
  high blood pressure. — 2nd ed.
  1. Hypertension
  I. Title
  616.1'32   RC685.H8

Library of Congress Cataloging in Publication Data
Hart, Julian Tudor.
  Hypertension: community control of high blood pressure.
  Includes index.
  1. Hypertension.   I. Title   [DNLM: 1. Hypertension.
WG 340 H325h]
RC685.H8H33   1980   616.1'32   87-8085

Produced by Longman Singapore Publishers (Pte) Ltd.
Printed in Singapore

To Mary, Robin, Rachel, Ben and all the other people of Glyncorrwg

The inquisitor: They say it is their mathematical tables and not the spirit of denial and doubt. But it is not their tables. A horrid unrest has come into the world. It is this unrest in their own brains which these men impose on the motionless earth. They cry, 'the figures compel us!', but whence come these figures? They come from doubt, as everyone knows. These men doubt everything. Are we to establish human society on doubt, and no longer on belief?

Bertolt Brecht — *Leben des Galilei*

Foreword to the First Edition

By any definition — and there are many of doubtful validity — hypertension is a common malady. It is also much in the public eye. In fact it is widely publicised in the United States as 'the silent killer', a title which adds greatly to the discomfiture of the patient. Naturally, therefore, there are many books by doctors dealing with either the condition as a whole or aspects of it. This book by Dr Julian Tudor Hart is the only one I know written by a primary care physician or family doctor for his colleagues. Since this is essentially a malady for family doctors this is a timely work.

The reader would expect the author to deal with the intellectual and technical aspects, such as causes, measurement of blood pressure and treatment. These things he will also find in other books, though perhaps not so lucidly expressed or so well balanced as here. What is, however, unique about this book is the account of how to manage the condition by a practitioner who is responsible for the whole field of human disease. In other words, how a generalist (be he physician or family doctor) can organise himself, his staff and his patients so that medical care can be of the highest efficiency and greatest efficacy. In doing this, Dr Tudor Hart shows unusual insight into patient behaviour. It is, of course, on such doctor–patient relationships that effective management depends. For the essential cause of failure of treatment is that in the early stages the patient feels perfectly well, and resents the nuisance of a regime which often makes him feel unwell. Avoidance of unnecessary restrictions, the choice by the doctor of the least unpleasant pills and an understanding by the patient of what the issue is for him are essential components of successful compliance.

Some years ago I wrote an obituary of that great Wensleydale practitioner, William Pickles. I quoted this from his work:

> And as I watched the evening train creeping up the valley
> with its pauses at our three stations, a quaint thought came

into my head and it was that there was hardly a man, woman or child in all those villages of whom I did not know the Christian name and with whom I was not on terms of intimate friendship. My wife and I say that we know most of the dogs and, indeed, some of the cats.

I would like to quote this from Dr Tudor Hart's book:

> For the past 18 years I have given day to day care to, and lived my own life among, a stable community of 1400 men and women of 20 years and over, for every one of whom I have known the mean of two or more casual pressures. From this I have learned that there is no feature of personality, physique, or other outward sign, that gives any clue to the pressures found on measurement. If psychosocial factors are important in determining blood pressure (and they probably are) they are too complex or remote in time from their consequences to be evident to observation alone. Such experience makes one impatient with simplistic hypotheses and single causes.

One of the most encouraging features of contemporary medicine in Britain is that the leaders of family doctors exhibit such wisdom and affection for their patients. It is a pleasure for an elderly physician like me to welcome younger men of such promise as Dr Julian Tudor Hart.

1980   Sir George Pickering

Preface

Since mid 1979, when the first edition of this book went to press, events have largely confirmed its general line, and the second edition can be simpler and less pretentious. Screening (or maximal case-finding) throughout the entire population at risk is now generally accepted as a necessary objective, and flexible, friendly, but positive systems of follow-up are recognised to be essential to effective control. The concept of high blood pressure as a reversible risk factor rather than a disease is generally accepted in words if not always in practice, and so are the conceptions of open negotiation with patients and continuity of personal care. Expansion of the primary care team with delegation of some responsibility for follow-up is accepted as necessary and inevitable. There have been important advances in drug treatment, more is known about the potential for harm as well as benefit from mass medication, and we are beginning to understand more about treatment without drugs. We are less ignorant about the multiple causes of primary hypertension, and have some firm ground at least on which to build plans for primary prevention.

I now also have 15 years of data on the management of a cohort of a 100% screened population aged 20–64 in 1968, when we first applied a blood pressure control policy to our entire community. This has been held on a mainframe computer at the Medical Research Council's clinical research centre at Northwick Park, and now that at last we have our own microcomputer in Glyncorrwg, it is beginning to be possible to use these data in patient care, rather than merely add to them. It is therefore possible to base the book on a little more documented evidence rather than gut-felt experience bolstered by an excessive number of references to other people's work.

The whole book has therefore been completely rewritten. I hope it will be useful to general practitioners and medical students, and to community physicians and hospital specialists who recognise the need for planned provision of secondary prevention services.

Chapter 10 from the first edition (Hypertension as a disease), of which I am fond, has been reprinted almost unchanged as Appendix VIII.

Colleagues who helped me in preparing the first edition were thanked there. For the second edition, I am indebted to Dr Paul Anand in Bombay and Professor John Milne in Johannesburg who took a lot of trouble providing information and references about hypertension in Indians and black South Africans, and to the authors and publishers who have agreed to reproduction of their illustrations. I am also grateful for continued help from my partner Dr Brian Gibbons, and to Drs Andy Haines, Graham Watt, Tom Meade and John Coope, to Chris Foy, and to the Glyncorrwg Health Centre service and research staff; Betty Ackery, Mair Boast, Catherine Edwards, Janet Jones, Margaret Jones, Evelyn Thomas, Margaret Thomas and Pam Walton. Finally, my publishers have remained patient despite a second edition long postponed.

May 1986   Julian Tudor Hart

Contents

1

Introduction

Hypertension presents the biggest single problem in continuing primary care. Depending on definitions and treatment policies, between 5 and 25% of the general adult population have blood pressures high enough to require some sort of medical intervention. In some urban black populations this proportion has been estimated to be as high as one-third of all adults.

To get some idea of the work involved in controlling this problem, it is useful to compare it with another common disorder, diabetes, which has a longer history of attempts at mass care. All forms of diabetes together affect only 2% of the population. Only about half of these cases are known, bringing effective demand down to 1%, and (in Britain) between one-half and two-thirds of these seem to be followed up in hospital outpatient clinics. These clinics are generally understaffed and overworked, and there is now fairly general agreement that specialist care is swamped with attempts to provide what should be routine primary care in a hospital setting. Safe and effective care in the community can be achieved where work is properly organised to provide it, but where it is not, traditional demand-led general practitioner (GP) care is neither safe nor effective. A controlled trial in Cardiff reported in 1984 that death rates in maturity-onset diabetics were three times higher in those allocated randomly to GP care than in those allocated to hospital outpatient care (Hayes & Harries 1984). The difference lay not in the skill, training, or dedication of these two groups of doctors, because they are in effect the same; routine hospital outpatient care of diabetics is mainly provided by junior doctors in training, more than half of whom will ultimately become GPs. The difference lies not in skill or conscience, but in the social organisation each is able to bring to the task; the hospital clinic is run by a team with division of labour and planned follow-up, with a system for recognising defaulters and chasing them up. No such system exists in the enormous majority of practices. The threefold difference in mortality revealed by the Cardiff trial shows the potential benefit of properly organised care even in the by no means optimal conditions of most hospital outpatient departments, and makes the current quality of care in general practice intolerable. We must do better; and it is *we* who must do it, because of the size of the problem, its clinical simplicity in all but a few cases, and the dependence of any solution on integration of care of non-insulin-dependent diabetes with the enormous range of other problems bound to occur in such vast numbers of people.

If recognised diabetes, affecting 1% of the population, is too big a task for our hospitals, how much more is this true of hypertension, affecting 5–25% of the population? Like the care of maturity-onset diabetes (and like most of the rest of medicine), effective care of 95% of hypertension consists of a few simple tasks applied consistently, honestly and imaginatively to the whole population at risk. It does require skills, but these are generally not of a very complex or technical nature, certainly nothing that cannot be taught in a short time to anyone encouraged to learn.

THE RULE OF HALVES

The rule of halves was first described by Wilber and Barrow in the USA, and remained true there until the early 1970s (Kannel et al 1981); half the hypertensives in the general population were not known, half of those known were not treated, and half of those treated were not controlled. It no longer applies in the USA, where overdiagnosis and overtreatment are now a bigger problem than underdiagnosis and undertreatment. By 1973–1974, only about a quarter of all hypertensives in the general US population were still undetected, and a quarter of those known were untreated. However, two-thirds of those treated were still uncontrolled, and 78% of black male hypertensives were undetected, untreated, or uncontrolled (Cowen et al 1981).

In Britain halves still rule. Studies in London (Kurji & Haines 1984; Michael 1984) and north-east Scotland (Ritchie & Currie 1983) showed that between one-third and one-half of all men over the age of 20 had no blood pressure recorded in their GP's notes over the previous 10 years, with no evidence of any recent improvement in recording. A survey of teaching practices in the Oxford region showed that only about half the middle-aged adults in these practice populations had any measurement of blood pressure recorded during the previous 10 years (Lawrence 1984).

DOES IT MATTER?

Doctors in the British National Health Service (NHS) have no incentive to diagnose or treat other than to meet consumer expectations (usually low and often inappropriate), and for the satisfaction of knowing they are doing their best to prevent the organ destruction which eventually follows most uncontrolled high blood pressure. Though these incentives are certainly substantial, they have evidently been insufficient so far to achieve the reorganisation of general practice necessary for complete, comprehensive and continuous care of this and other common chronic disorders.

A study of medical deaths in hospital in England and Scotland (Whitfield 1981) showed that of 105 patients who died under 50 years of age from complications of hypertension, in about one-quarter the disease had never been recognised, in another quarter it had never been treated, and in the remaining half it had been treated but not controlled. Hypertension had been both recognised and controlled in only 2% of these 105 hypertensives. General practice is, on the whole, hard work, and laziness is not the problem. The most exhausting thing about general practice is the futility of much of the work many of us still do, a custom-geared treadmill of frequent but ineffective consultations giving superficial attention to symptoms but showing little concern with causes. There is now fairly general understanding that hypertension presents an unusually favourable opportunity to do effective work which can reduce the burden of illness and early death; but the response has to be organised. It is not just a question of the same old people working in the same old way, but harder. To suggest that it is is divisive, and plays into the hands of those who believe that public services can expand production without real investment.

Control of high blood pressure before the onset of organ damage is an exercise in prevention of disease, not its treatment. As our entire tradition of general practice lies in a demand-led response to symptoms and we are paid and organised accordingly, it should not be surprising that we are better at responding to wants than at searching for needs. No one, no doctor, no Government, not even any Treasury official would deny the need to provide some kind of service for the victims of stroke, a consequence of untreated hypertension which is itself almost untreatable; but the task of organising an effective *preventive* service still depends almost entirely on the initiative of individual GPs who are prepared, against all fashionable trends, to regard their work as a public service rather than a private business. The continued high incidence of stroke, retinal and renal damage, acute and chronic heart failure, multi-infarct dementia, and the many other preventable complications of hypertension, are clear evidence that a more active policy which would encourage more practices to organise, set objectives, and measure their attainment is long overdue.

Using data from the Royal College of General Practitioners' (RCGP) second national morbidity survey, Robson (1986) showed that just to record blood pressure once every 5 years in people aged 45–64, and to follow up the borderline and hypertensive patients once a year would require GPs (or other primary health workers) to undertake 286 per 1000 more consultations a year, compared with the 636 per 1000 now done in this age-group. This would represent a 45% increase in workload, if done with present practice organisation.

I do not believe that the big changes required in general practice to manage this and other common chronic disorders can be safely, effectively or economically operated through market forces; that is, through fee-paid episodic service, competing with other personal costs. That results only in creating an uncontrolled market above whatever intervention threshold medical credulity allows, in which GPs become as biased toward overdiagnosis and overtreatment as we have hitherto been to passivity. Nor do I believe we should follow the corporate solutions offered by the Health Maintenance Organizations in the USA, in which doctors have become salaried cogs in the wheels of a profitable medical–industrial complex. British general practice is still not far beyond a cottage industry, but we already have most of the structures essential to the local planning, control, and accountability essential for effective primary care in a democratic society. The management of hypertension in whole local populations could be one good way of learning to plan the conservation of health democratically at a neighbourhood level, a process which will eventually be recognised as essential for all common disorders.

STARTING FROM WHERE WE ARE, WITH THE PEOPLE WE HAVE

British GPs have one huge advantage over most of our colleagues in other countries; we know who our patients are. Our populations are registered and listed, so that we can plan their care if we really want to. Though patients can change their GP if they wish, few do so, and they cannot take themselves off to consult specialists in hospitals, or specialoids outside them, without referral through their GP. Patients do not pay a consulting fee, so we have a free hand in organising follow-up. Prescription charges are now a real impediment to treatment in my experience, having risen by 1000% (at the time of writing) since the accession to power of our present Government; even so, they apply to only 15% of the population (though the proportion must be more for middle-aged hypertensives), and the £2.20 charge is still a lot less than the real cost of most though not all antihypertensive drugs. The capitation payment system encourages GPs to do a little for a lot of people rather than a lot for a few people. In some ways, this may be surprisingly well suited to the management of hypertension.

SIX ORGANISATIONAL QUESTIONS FOR WHOLE COMMUNITY CARE

Whatever care system they work in, family doctors have to find answers to six sets of organisational questions if they want to control high blood pressure on a community scale:

1. How to identify the population at risk. Even inner city populations are more stable than most of us think. Of those randomly selected for study in the huge Hypertension Detection and Follow-up Program in the USA (mainly in central urban populations) 11% changed address within 2 years, but only 4% moved outside the area of their health care facility.
2. How to be sure that all the adults in this defined population have blood pressures measured and recorded at regular intervals.
3. How to use these measurements to divide the population into three treatment categories:

   a follow and treat;
   b follow and observe;
   c recheck after an interval.

4. How to organise follow-up, maintain compliance in treated cases, and establish some kind of supervision for those observed but not treated.
5. How to integrate control of hypertension with management

of other problems, and co-ordinate care with other agencies.

6. How to train patients, staff, and doctors themselves in the new and different ways of thinking and acting required for an effective search for needs, as well as response to symptoms.

Most of this book will discuss these six problems.

REFERENCES

Cowan L, Detels R, Farber M et al 1980 Residential mobility and long-term treatment of hypertension. Journal of Community health 5:159

Hayes T M, Harries T J 1984 Randomised controlled trial of routine hospital clinic care versus routine general practice care for type II diabetes. British Medical Journal 289:728

Kannel W B, Wolf P A, McGee D L et al 1981 Systolic blood pressure, arterial rigidity and the risk of stroke. Journal of the American Medical Association 245:1225

Kurji K H, Haines A P 1984 Detection and management of hypertension in general practices in northwest London. British Medical Journal 288:903

Lawrence M S 1984 Hypertension in general practice. British Medical Journal 288:1156

Michael G 1984 Quality of care in managing hypertension by case-finding in northwest London. British Medical Journal 288:906

Ritchie L D, Currie A M 1983 Blood pressure recording by general practitioners in northwest Scotland. British Medical Journal 286:107

Robson J 1986 Bridging the expectation-delivery gap: can it be left to chance? In: Gray D P (ed) The medical annual. John Wright, Bristol, pp 197–205

Whitfield A G W 1981 Young medical deaths: their cause and prevention. Update (London) 1249–1254

2

Internal mechanisms and some mechanisms of secondary hypertension

Despite the predictive power of mean arterial pressure over many years ahead, the level of arterial pressure has immediate biological meaning only through the effect it has on perfusion through the terminal capillary loop. This is one of the great biological constants: a constant inflow pressure of 32 mmHg (a little more than the colloid osmotic pressure of plasma) and an outflow pressure of 15 mmHg (a little below it).

This pressure gradient has to be maintained throughout an extraordinarily variable capillary network. Total blood flow at rest is about 6/l min, of which 13% goes to brain, 24% to gut, 19% to kidneys, 4% to heart muscle, and 21% to voluntary muscle. During maximal exercise brain flow stays the same, total blood flow increases more than fourfold to 25/l min, gut flow falls nearly fivefold, kidney flow falls fourfold, heart muscle flow increases fourfold, and flow through voluntary muscle increases 18-fold. None of this seems to be any different in hypertensive subjects, until they begin to go into heart failure.

In the most general terms, biological control systems operate at three levels; rapid responses through the nervous system, delayed responses through hormone systems, and long-term adaptation through modification of the composition, structure, and behaviour of any or all systems, organs and tissues. Again in the most general terms, each of these three involves a sequence of control systems, so that if one fails, a back-up system operates at a more primitive level. By the nature of its techniques, experimental physiology has first revealed the crudest and most primitive systems that are least relevant to the intact patient at an early stage of disorder. It is easier to study short-term, rapidly reversible mechanisms than long-term adaptations, so we know more about them, though they are probably less relevant to the natural history of hypertension in real populations.

A CRUDE MODEL

As every elementary medical scholar knows,

Arterial pressure = heart output × peripheral resistance

Both heart output and arteriolar constriction are under autonomic control, with cortical connections. The effects of alarm on heart rate and stroke volume, and its rather smaller effects on arterial pressure, are well known, but these are short-term effects which may or may not be relevant to a sustained rise in pressure.

There is some still rather contradictory but on the whole persuasive evidence that primary hypertension starts with a phase of high output, possibly initiated by a state of chronic alarm. By the time high blood pressure is clinically recognisable this is no longer the case, and the immediate mechanism of hypertension is peripheral resistance raised by narrowed arterioles. Initially this is caused only by contraction of the muscle layer and is fully reversible. Later, usually many years later, it may also be caused by arteriolar and arterial damage, with deposition of fibrin which then organises to cholesterol plaque, and is no longer fully reversible. The rate and extent of this process seem to depend both on the level of arterial pressure already attained (so that high blood pressure becomes itself a cause of higher pressure, a self-accelerating cycle) and on the level of blood cholesterol. Atheroma is not a necessary part of this process, because severe hypertension, with consequent stroke or left ventricular failure, is common in populations with mean total cholesterol levels below 4.00 mmol (155 mg)/dl, for example in some black South African and Japanese communities, in whom atheroma and coronary disease are virtually unknown. In our culture, atheroma usually modifies the course of hypertension, often eventually leading to falling output from an ischaemic heart, with a consequent fall in arterial pressure, providing the patient has not already succumbed to coronary disease.

So there is evidence, again not always consistent, that primary hypertension conforms to the following crude sequential model, at least in our kind of society:

Rising heart output →
Functionally raised peripheral resistance →
Structurally raised peripheral resistance →
Falling heart output

INITIATING MECHANISMS

If, and this is by no means certain, sustained rise in blood pressure is usually preceded by high output, what initiates that rise?

Until recently there were two fairly well defined schools of thought, the stressites and the saltites. Few would deny that at least some kinds of stress, and some levels of dietary sodium, have some effect on hypertension at some point in its development, and are possible or probable external causes; there is more about both these causes in Chapter 3. Here they must be briefly discussed as initiators of different sets of internal mechanisms.

Stress and enhanced positive autonomic feedback

Until about ten years ago, this was certainly the most favoured theory of causation for what was then called essential hypertension. Depending mainly on differences in personality and life experience, it was postulated that some people were more liable than others to convert normal, transient hypertensive responses to current stress into sustained hypertensive responses to stress no longer present, perhaps through some intermediate process whereby structural changes in the kidney or arterioles made the process irreversible. This was translated clinically into early labile and later fixed hypertension. The internal mechanism for this sequence was autonomic response to stress signals from the brain cortex leading to increased arteriolar tone. An apparently good animal model was found in the Wistar rat, which became hypertensive when overcrowded or tormented in various ways, unless it was protected before maturity by blockade of its autonomic beta-receptors.

Though attractive, and still commanding a mass following, this theory has not stood up well to critical experiment with human subjects, nor does it provide consistent explanations for epidemiological findings.

Sodium overload and impaired negative renal feedback

This theory postulates that arterial pressure is normally controlled by a negative feedback system, in which raised pressure leads to diuresis and a fall in blood volume. Hypertension is caused by dietary sodium overload, followed by a rise in renal threshold for diuresis, leading to expanded blood volume. This is a credible hypothesis since dietary sodium in industrialised societies, at a daily intake of 130–400 mmol, is vastly greater than the minimum physiological intake of 10 mmol/day, at which level nobody gets either hypertension or any rise in blood pressure with age.

Again, suitable strains of rat exist which respond to sodium overload by developing lethal hypertension; but attempts to show an increase in blood volume in early hypertension in humans, or in the pre-hypertensive offspring of hypertensive parents, have generally failed. Blood pressure falls in everyone with severe sodium depletion to intakes of 10 mmol/day or less, but more tolerable reductions of dietary sodium to around 80–100 mmol daily have little if any effect on borderline hypertension, a modest effect on moderate hypertension, and a marked effect only on fairly severe hypertension, suggesting that responsiveness to sodium depletion is linked to the effects of high arterial pressure rather than its cause.

Inheritance

Genetic theory has been used to plug some of the holes in these two leaky arguments. If predictions made from intensive laboratory studies of small numbers of patients cannot be confirmed in large population samples, one explanation might be that hypertensive mechanisms apply only to a subset of genetically susceptible people.

High blood pressure runs in families. The better you know your population, the more striking this truth becomes. I have not been able to find anyone in Glyncorrwg with severe hypertension (diastolic pressure >120 mmHg) whose parents' blood pressures were known, in whom one or both parents were not hypertensive (diastolic pressure >100mmHg). It is now universally accepted that hypertension cannot be inherited through a single gene, but polygenic inheritance is the best single predictor of individual pressures in industrialised populations, showing a regression coefficient of 0.34 for first-degree relatives of both sexes at all levels of pressure (Miall & Oldham 1955, 1958). This means that about two-thirds of the variability within such a population is accounted for by inheritance. A more practical conclusion is that inheritance determines internal mechanisms through which external causes can operate selectively, in some but not all of a population.

Sex

Published studies of hypertension from general practice and hospital clinical series have always shown a large excess of women.

Epidemiological studies of whole populations, on the other hand, have always shown an excess of male hypertensives up to 45–50 years of age, after which a female excess gradually builds up with increasing age. Because the Framingham study began at age 45, it has not contributed data on blood pressure in young adults. There is a large male excess in young hypertensives, which we have found consistently in the fully screened population of Glyncorrwg. This has been strikingly confirmed by the Medical Research Council (MRC) national birth cohort study, which showed that high blood pressure (>140/90 mmHg) was almost twice as common in young men as in young women (Wadsworth et al 1985).

Disorders of cell membrane ion transport

First in the 1950s, and accelerating through the 1970s, a completely new approach to causation began to challenge previous assumptions that the mechanism of hypertension must be a failure at some local point in one of several control systems. This was a search for differences in transport of sodium ion across cell membranes in both directions, initially in renal and vascular tissues, later extended to all tissues including red blood cells, which were easier to sample and handle in the laboratory. The subject has been well summarised by Postnov and Orlov (1984).

As usual, what at first promised to be a simple solution has since proved contradictory and confusing. Even the methodology is still in dispute, and early attempts to apply still unstandardised laboratory techniques to small, poorly defined samples with various alleged genetic characteristics have failed to give replicable results. Attention has moved beyond the behaviour of sodium ion to studies of potassium and calcium ion, with attempts to link these with dietary and genetic differences. Stamler's group in Chicago has taken the (as far as I know) unique step of applying ion transport measurements to adequately defined population samples (Cooper et al 1984). They found convincing evidence of small but significant differences in sodium transport across cell membranes between hypertensive and normotensive subjects drawn from the same population. They also found evidence of systematic differences between adolescent offspring of hypertensive and normotensive parents (Cooper et al 1983).

This field is promising and important. Once the methodology becomes standardised, and researchers agree on a more plausible pace for innovative theory, we can expect exciting results. For the time being, we must leave it to the small band of experts who understand both its possibilities and its limitations.

SOME MECHANISMS OF SECONDARY HYPERTENSION

The main clinical problem with the fewer than 2% of hypertensives for which a classical cause can be found is to look for them effectively and intelligently, with a reasonable use of diagnostic resources. This problem is considered in Chapter 12. Here we are concerned with them as examples of internal mechanisms.

Coarctation

Coarctation, a stricture of the aorta usually close to the entry point of the ductus arteriosus, but occasionally in the abdominal aorta above or below the renal arteries, probably but not certainly begins with a prenatal malformation. The mechanism of hypertension in this case seems deceptively obvious; mechanical obstruction to perfusion of the lower half of the body requires a large increase in left ventricular output, with high arterial pressure in the upper limbs and low pressure in the lower limbs. As usual, it's not that simple. Hypertension often persists after reconstruction of the stricture, showing once again that initiating causes are not the same as maintaining causes, and that high arterial pressure seems to cause adaptive changes which are in turn a cause of yet higher pressure. Reduced perfusion of the kidneys may be an important secondary cause.

Renal hypertension

More than 90% of all classical secondary hypertension is renal in origin. Evidence on mechanisms for this is conflicting, but is on the whole consistent with the view that if structural damage to the kidney, whatever its cause, raises arterial pressure, it does so by causing renal ischaemia, provoking secretion of renin and thus activating plasma substrate to yield angiotensin, the most potent vasocontrictor substance known. Renin release is normally reactive to dietary sodium intake, not ischaemia, but there is some evidence that at a very early stage in reduction of renal arterial flow, renin release is increased, perhaps initiating a rise in blood pressure which is maintained later by other mechanisms. Virtually all forms of renal damage may do this: obstructive, inflammatory, infective, neoplastic, and traumatic.

Bilateral causes

The commonest form of renal damage is chronic infection leading to scarring, and which is usually bilateral. Infection without scarring, acute or chronic, has no effect on pressure. In girls aged 5–12, about 12 per 1000 have chronic or recurrent bacteriuria detectable by dipculture, and of these about half have radiologically demonstrable abnormalities of the urinary tract, with vesico-ureteric reflux alone in roughly half of these, and reflux plus scarring in the other half; it is this last group which may go on to develop chronic pyelonephritis with raised arterial pressure (Asscher 1983). Prevalence in boys is still unknown, but is certainly much less. Unfortunately it seems that once the scarring process begins, it is irreversible; long-term antibiotic control of infection seems to make no difference. The treatable stage of vesico-ureteric reflux is probably between birth and 4 or 5 years of age, and diagnostic screening should probably be concentrated on this age group, which really means that GPs should do it by systematic use of dip-cultures in suspicious (usually minor) illness, picking up the occasional cases of surgically correctable obstructive lesions at the same time.

In primary care, the next most frequent problem of this kind is the diabetic kidney, which is associated with hypertension in 90% of cases. This is a common and, at an early stage, treatable and probably preventable cause of eventual end-stage renal failure. It seems to be relentlessly progressive by the time a clinically detectable proteinuria is present, but if control of diabetes is optimal and if hypertension is assiduously controlled, the rate of deterioration of renal function may be delayed sufficiently to allow a normal lifespan.

Gouty nephropathy is another less frequent cause of both hypertension and renal failure, important because it often presents with recurrent stone treated by surgeons rather than physicians. GPs may find themselves the only physicians in the mix, and unless they show some clinical curiosity, nobody does, and the underlying abnormality may continue uncorrected.

Acute and chronic glomerulonephritis, much rarer now than before the demise of the Streptococcus after the Second World War, are other bilateral causes of renal hypertension, probably initiated by renal ischaemia caused by autoimmune vasculitis. Unless it is controlled, this hypertension then accelerates further renal damage, leading ultimately to end-stage renal failure.

The adult form of polycystic kidneys runs in families as a simple

Mendelian dominant, and may therefore be locally common. The kidneys are radiologically normal until late childhood. Hypertension develops in about 80% of cases, but is rarely severe. As always, hypertension accelerates deterioration in renal function and therefore needs assiduous control.

Unilateral causes

Ever since the Goldblatt kidney, students have been loaded with simplistic physiology and warnings about the critical importance of detecting unilateral renal disease causing secondary hypertension, the favourite model being unilateral renal artery stenosis. Other causes are renin-secreting tumours, other renal tumours both benign and malignant, unilateral chronic pyelitis and hydronephrosis and renal tuberculosis.

Stenosis or occlusion of a renal artery is said to be the commonest form of unilateral renal disease causing ischaemic secondary hypertension, possibly accounting for up to 4% of all hypertensives, about 200 000 people in the whole of Britain. As clinical and autopsy studies show renal artery stenosis in up to 46% of normotensives, it is difficult to guess what, if anything, these figures mean (Mackay et al 1983). Renal artery stenoses do not behave in the relatively simple fashion found by Goldblatt in his dogs. Yet again, initiating causes and maintaining causes are different, so hypertension frequently persists even after stenosis is relieved. Even a prospective series of nephrectomies for unilateral chronic pyelonephritis before the onset of hypertension has shown no prophylactic effect (Asscher 1983).

Phaeochromocytoma

These usually benign tumours are very rare, but important to find because they may cause disabling symptoms for many years, which are often missed. Many of them are familial, with autosomal dominant inheritance with high penetrance. About 1% of patients with neurofibromatosis develop these tumours, of which 90% arise in the adrenal medulla, but they may be anywhere where there is chromaffin tissue. All secrete noradrenaline (norepinephrine), which is the cause of hypertension if and when this occurs. They may also produce adrenaline (epinephrine), which reduces diastolic pressure, and both the precursors and degradation products of catecholamines in various proportions, causing a wide variety of symptoms. The hypertension caused by these tumours is not always paroxysmal, and rarely severe.

Primary aldosteronism

This probably has a prevalence of between 0.1 and 1% of all hypertensives. In classical Conn's syndrome aldosterone is secreted from a benign tumour of the adrenal medulla, but similar effects on arterial pressure occur if there is autonomous hypersecretion from an apparently normal adrenal, or from adrenal or ovarian carcinoma. Hypertension is invariably present, but is seldom severe. It seems to be caused by the sequence:

excess aldosterone → K depletion
Na retention → raised plasma volume, high cardiac output and low renin

Intracranial tumours

Lesions causing raised intracranial pressure can present as fairly severe hypertension, often intermittent, and the accompanying headache, papilloedema and central nervous system (CNS) signs can be confusing. Experimentally, electric stimulation of the frontal and temporal cortex and the floor of the fourth ventricle cause a rise in arterial pressure. Posterior fossa tumours are particularly likely to cause hypertension, probably by distorting the brain stem.

Cushing's syndrome and hypothyroidism

Hypertension occurs in about three-quarters of all cases of Cushing's syndrome, which seems to have roughly the same prevalence as phaeochromocytoma and hyperaldosteronism. The chief mechanism of the hypertension seems to be the sequence:

excess cortisol → increased angiotension substrate

Hypertension is 50–100% commoner than in the general population in both symptomatic and biochemical hypothyroidism (Bing & Swales 1983). The mechanism is unknown. Hypothyroidism is usually associated with raised total serum cholesterol, but the large excess of coronary disease in these people occurs almost entirely in those with hypertension. In about half of these, pressure returns to normal after correction of the thyroid deficiency.

Laboratory methods on a population scale

The two classical contending theories, and their more sophisticated descendants and combinations, have been excellently reviewed by Stevo Julius, in a paper recommended to anyone interested in the research end of this field (Julius et al 1983). He argues that no causal hypothesis can be convincingly supported by studies either of large numbers of laboratory rats, or of the very small numbers of human subjects hitherto subjected to sophisticated and invasive laboratory tests. Nor can this be done by large-scale epidemiological studies of the traditional kind, which apply simple, non-invasive measurements to large representative populations. We shall not get any convincing answers until these two hitherto separate methods of study are combined, and more sophisticated techniques are applied to very much larger, more carefully sampled groups of people, followed over years rather than weeks or months. Why not through general practice?

REFERENCES

Asscher A W 1983 Urinary tract infection as a cause of hypertension in man. In: Robertson J I S (ed), Handbook of hypertension vol 2: clinical aspects of secondary hypertension. Elsevier Science Publishers, Oxford, pp 18, 29
Bing R F, Swales J D 1983 Thyroid disease and hypertension. In: Robertson J I S (ed) Handbook of hypertension vol 2: clinical aspects of secondary hypertension, Elsevier Science Publishers, Oxford, p 276
Cooper R, Miller K, Trevisan M et al 1983 Family history of hypertension and red cell cation transport in high school students. Journal of Hypertension 1:145
Cooper R, Trevisan M, Ostrow D et al 1984 Blood pressure and sodium–lithium countertransport: findings in population-based surveys. Journal of Hypertension 2:467
Julius S, Weder A B, Egan B M 1983 Pathophysiology of early hypertension: implications for epidermiologic research. In: Gross F, Strasser T (eds) Mild hypertension: recent advances. Raven Press, New York, p 219
MacKay A, Brown J J, Lever A F et al 1983 Unilateral renal disease in hypertension. In: Robertson J I S (ed) Handbook of hypertension vol 2: clinical aspects of secondary hypertension. Elsevier Science Publishers, Oxford, p 35
Miall W E, Oldham P D 1955 A study of arterial blood pressure and its inheritance in a sample of the general population. Clinical Science 14:459
Miall W M, Oldham P D 1958 Factors influencing arterial pressure in the general population. Clinical Science 17:409
Postnov Y V, Orlov S N 1984 Cell membrane alteration as a source of primary hypertension. Journal of Hypertension 2:1
Wadsworth M E J, Cripps H A, Midwinter R E et al 1985 Blood pressure in a national birth cohort at the age of 36 related to social and family factors, smoking, and body mass. British Medical Journal 291:1534

3

External causes

Discussing causation of primary hypertension in 1954, Pickering's group concluded:

> . . .what has been called essential hypertension is a purely arbitrary segregation of those having arterial pressures in the higher ranges and having no disease to which these high pressures can be attributed. The factors concerned in the pathogenesis of so-called essential hypertension are thus those concerned in determining the arterial pressure in the population at large. (Hamilton et al 1954)

An example of a distribution of blood pressures in the general population is shown in Figure 3.1. Wherever total populations are studied in industrialised societies, similar distributions are found, unimodal and skewed to the right (more highs than lows). They also show a consistent rise in group mean pressure and increasing skewness with age (Fig. 3.2; Hamilton et al 1954).

The search for causes of high blood pressure should begin with the study of these differences throughout their range, throughout life, and in different environments and societies. Then we can ask two important questions:

1. Why, in some populations but not others, is there a positively skewed distribution within age-groups and a rise with age? Or, why are there between-population differences?
2. Why, within national populations with the usual positively skewed and age-related distribution, do mean pressures vary so much from one population to another? Or, why are there within-population differences?

We may then begin to identify external and therefore avoidable causes, as well as internal and possibly treatable mechanisms, both of which can be experimentally verified.

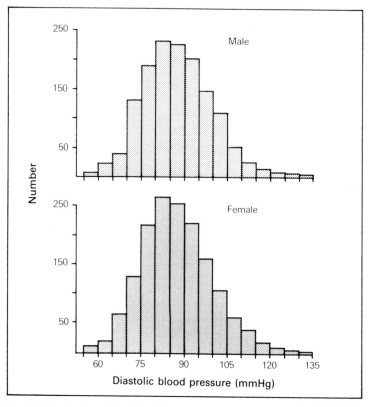

Fig. 3.1 Distribution of diastolic blood pressure in 4500 men and women aged 45–64 in Scotland (Hawthorne et al 1974).

AGE AND SENESCENCE

Populations have been found in South America, Africa and the Pacific in whom arterial pressure remains low throughout life. Common features of all of them are persistence of a New Stone Age culture, very low sodium intakes (10–30 mmol daily), high potassium intakes, low body fat, and high energy expenditure with relatively low energy intake. When migrants from these populations move to industrialised societies, group mean arterial pressures rise, hypertension appears at one end of the distribution, and blood pressures rise with age. Where they adopt diets in which animal fats account for 35–40% or more of energy intake (for example, Japanese migrants to the USA), hypertension begins to operate as

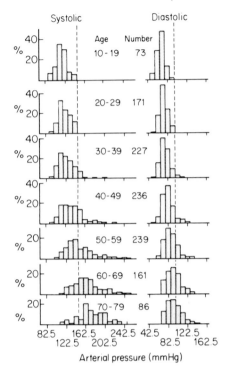

Fig. 3.2 Frequency distribution of systolic and diastolic blood pressure for females of the population sample arranged by age in decades. The histogram shows the percentages having a given range of pressure. Since in the range of pressure 50–59 mmHg there were only two sets of readings, at 50 and 55 mmHg, the centre of this range has been shown as the mean of the two readings, namely, at 52.5 mmHg, and similarly throughout the blood pressure scale. The numbers of subjects in each decade are shown in the centre. Dashed lines have been drawn to indicate the commonest current practice of distinguishing between normal pressure and hypertension, the latter including systolic pressures of 150 mmHg or over and diastolic pressures of 100 mmHg or over. It will be seen that there is no natural division at this or any other line (Hamilton et al 1954). (from: Pickering, G. W. *High Blood Pressure, 2nd edition*, Churchill Livingstone, 1968)

a risk factor for coronary disease as well as heart failure and stroke, and coronary deaths become common. Where intake of animal fats remains low (as in native Japanese and black South Africans), hypertensive heart failure and stroke become common, but coronary heart disease remains rare, even if (as in both these examples) people smoke heavily.

So although even in childhood age has a closer positive association with arterial pressure than weight or height, this association is not causal. Inevitably and inextricably, age is composed of both time and experience; evidently it is the experience, rather than lapsed time, which joins with polygenic inheritance to determine the distribution of blood pressure.

SODIUM INTAKE

Hypertension does not exist where sodium intakes are less than 30 mmol daily. Stroke, a common sequel to severe hypertension, is exceptionally common in countries like Portugal and northern Japan, where sodium intakes are unusually high: more than 400 mmol/day. Sodium intakes in Britain are generally around 130–160 mmol/day, rather less than Australia and the USA which have average daily intakes around 200 mmol.

In 1954 Dahl bred a strain of rats that became hypertensive when they were made to eat enormous quantities of salt, and another strain which did not become hypertensive no matter how much salt they were given. He thought there was a similar genetic difference in humans, and that the principal cause of primary hypertension was the unnecessarily sodium–rich diet of all fully developed cultures. There is now yet another strain of rat which shows a fall in blood pressure when overfed with salt to the same improbable extent as Dahl's strain. There is a fairly low limit to what we can learn from other species.

Evidence that sodium restriction is an effective method of treatment of high blood pressure is discussed in Chapter 14. Here we are concerned only with whether it is an important initiating or maintaining cause.

There is powerful circumstantial evidence in favour of sodium overload as an initiating cause, mainly the differences between populations already referred to. However, there are many other differences between generally underfed New Stone Age populations and those in more developed economies; a notable example is the marked obesity of migrant Polynesians in New Zealand, compared with skinny, low-salt Pacific islanders. Many of the original studies on which the salt argument is based used crude methods to estimate sodium intake, and blood pressure measurements were often poorly performed. Many were based on superficial assessment of diet, without measurement of urinary sodium output, or in hot climates where loss of sodium in sweat makes measurement more difficult. Even when such measurements were done, many were based on casual samples of urine. Day-to-day variability of sodium intake, in developed societies at least, is so great that within-subject variability is greater than between-subject variability for 24-h urine collections, and reliable characterisation of habitual individual intake probably requires continuous and complete collections of urine over at least 7 days. Hardly any of the original studies meet these criteria, and few of the more recent ones (Watt & Foy 1982). This difficulty will be overcome when the international multicentre World Health Organization study Intersalt reports in a few years' time.

Hofman et al (1983) showed a small but significant positive association between blood pressure and sodium intake in newborn infants. Stamler's group first showed a similar very small positive association in older children, but was unable to replicate this in a larger population (Cooper et al 1983). Very large-scale and methodologically sound studies of adults have failed to show any positive association between sodium intake (measured as output) and arterial pressure (Kesteloot & Geboers 1982). Here in Glyncorrwg, a double-blind randomised control study of two genetic groups from the same population, offspring of parents who both had blood pressures in the top third of the population distribution, and offspring of parents who both had blood pressures in the bottom third of the distribution, showed no fall in pressure in either group despite a reduction in sodium intake to below 50 mmol/day sustained for 4 weeks (Watt et al 1985). There was also no difference in sodium intake between the same contrasting genetic groups when they were left to choose their own preferred diet (Watt et al 1983), so the idea of genetically determined salt avidity was not supported.

It is likely, though not proven, that if sodium intake were reduced to a level between the physiological minimum, around 10 mmol/day; and the highest levels found in communities which have no hypertension, around 30 mmol/day, high blood pressure would either disappear or become very rare. There are advocates of this policy, and some of them even claim to enjoy such a diet. Having tried it myself, I cannot agree that this will be a feasible policy for primary prevention in the foreseeable future; perhaps everyone should try it (with measured sodium outputs) before stating an opinion.

The real argument is not about such drastic reductions to achieve an unrecognisably different diet, but the effect of reductions of about one-third, say from 150 to 100 mmol sodium daily. Despite the poor, indeed still weakening evidence for the theory of sodium overload, there is still strong circumstantial evidence in its favour, and it remains attractive. It is still possible that there is a critical threshold much higher than the 80–100 mmol/day target arbitrarily chosen for most intervention studies, possibly more relevent to the very high intakes of Japan and Portugal than to the British mean daily intake of around 150 mmol. It is also possible that there is some critical period in childhood or adolescence during which sodium overload has a lasting effect.

INTAKE OF POTASSIUM, FAT AND VEGETARIAN DIET

There is now fairly consistent evidence that an increase in potassium intake of about 30%, or a fall in the Na/K ratio of food (measured as 24-h urine output) has a lowering effect on blood pressure, and that (in contrast to similar studies of sodium) arterial pressure in populations correlates negatively with K output, and positively with Na/K ratio (Langford 1983). All very low-sodium populations are also high-potassium populations, reflecting intakes of cereals, fruit and vegetables, which may at least partly explain the generally lower pressures found in vegetarians (Rouse & Beilin 1984). Precise dietary studies are extremely difficult, with numerous confounding factors both in the food itself, and in associated features such as religiosity or attitudes to alcohol, and it is usually impossible to do them blindly with valid controls. There is fairly convincing evidence that animal fats raise blood pressure (Puska et al 1983), and their absence may have a share in the vegetarian effect.

These studies need to be confirmed, but already they fit in well with the wealth of evidence that reduction of animal fat and increase in fibre reduce total blood cholesterol and the risk of coronary disease in populations, whatever their effect on blood pressure.

OBESITY

Obesity can be most easily expressed as body mass index (BMI = metric weight/metric height squared). From a BMI of about 30.0, death rates increase steeply, mainly from cancer, coronary disease and stroke. The association is complex. Obesity has little independent effect on coronary mortality until it is fairly severe, and there is consistent evidence that although obesity in childhood and youth is a predictor of future hypertension (Wadsworth et al

1983), thin hypertensives have a higher mortality than fat hypertensives when standardised for blood pressure (Connor & Khaw 1985). These effects are real, and not caused by the artefacts associated with use of a short sphygmomanometer cuff on a fat arm. There is some evidence that fat bellies are more important than fat arms and legs. A convenient way of measuring this central obesity is to divide metric belly circumference by hip circumference; Bjorntorp (1985) has shown that coronary risk increases steeply when this coefficient exceeds 1.000.

Weight reduction (mean loss 4 kg) alone did not reduce blood pressure in an excellent controlled trial in men, at mean age 46 years (Haynes et al 1984). Whether weight reduction might have prevented later hypertension in much younger subjects, say in their early 20s, is an important question on which there is as yet no evidence.

Together with sodium overload, adolescent and young adult

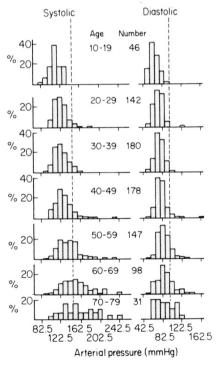

Fig. 3.3 Frequency distribution of systolic and diastolic blood pressure for males. (from: Pickering, G. W. *High Blood Pressure, 2nd edition* Churchill Livingstone, 1968).

obesity and alcohol are probably the prime suspects as mass causes for primary hypertension.

ALCOHOL

Numerous population studies have shown a positive linear association between systolic and diastolic blood pressure and alcohol consumption (Arkwright et al 1982).

In October 1985, an audit of 71 male hypertensives identified by screening and currently being followed up in Glyncorrwg showed 17 (24%) with recognised alcohol problems either past or present, compared with 69 out of 580 (12%) for the adult male population as a whole. None of the 61 hypertensive women had a known alcohol problem, compared with 16 out of 606 adult women (3%).

Clinically, it is a common observation that otherwise refractory hypertension often comes under control when heavy drinking is recognised and controlled. However, puritan zeal should be tempered by equally consistent evidence that people who drink not more than two or three units of alcohol daily (1 unit = 1 glass of wine, half a pint of beer, or 1 measure of spirits) have lower coronary risks than either teetotalers or heavier drinkers, probably because of an effect on HDL cholesterol.

SMOKING

Cigarette smoking has a brief hypertensive effect of no consequence to long-term pressures, which in most population studies are slightly lower in smokers. It has a dramatic effect on coronary risk, with a threefold increase in middle-aged male hypertensive smokers compared with hypertensive non-smokers (Samuelsson et al 1985), and there is good evidence that it may precipitate malignant hypertension in young women on the oral contraceptive pill (Petitti & Klatsky 1983).

ENVIRONMENTAL STRESS

Pain, anger, curiosity, fear, excitement, and embarrassment all cause a transient rise in blood pressure in everyone. It is reasonable to suppose that sustained repetition of these feelings, or the circumstances that give rise to them, are a cause, even *the* cause, of sustained high blood pressure. Consistent evidence to support this idea, however, has been difficult to find.

This evidence could be of two kinds: prospective evidence of more pressor events, or of greater pressor response to an equal burden of events, in early hypertensives than in normotensive controls. At the rather crude level at which these ideas were originally expressed (and which still grip the imaginations of nearly all patients and most doctors), there is little hard evidence to support either of them; however, subtler forms of internalised stress remain likely (Henry 1980), though rather difficult to test. It is perhaps surprising that the aggressive Type A personality of Rosenman and Friedman, shown to be an important predictor for coronary heart disease in white collar but not blue collar workers in the USA (but not in Britain), shows no association with blood pressure in population samples (Shekelle et al 1976; Haynes et al 1978).

A third kind of evidence would be controlled trials of stress reduction in hypertensives, as a method of treatment. Such trials are extremely difficult to carry out, but some of their results are now very persuasive. These are discussed at length in Chapter 14.

Much more is now known about measurable markers of autonomic activity, and the many pitfalls in their interpretation. Studies of the kind urged by Julius, referred to in Chapter 2, are now urgently needed, combining sophisticated laboratory methods with rigorous epidemiological design, and applied to larger populations.

SKIN COLOUR AND SOCIAL CLASS

Data from the USA have consistently shown higher blood pressure levels for blacks than whites, and much higher levels of mortality from stroke and heart failure. Differences between blacks and whites in plasma renin, response to diuretics and to beta-blockers, and in cell membrane ion transport, have usually been interpreted as additional evidence in favour of a 'racial' difference in susceptibility to hypertension. Since in evolutionary terms a black skin represents remote origins in a hot, dry, and often salt-deficient environment, some of these differences are biologically plausible.

However, again there are difficulties. Studies of black, white, and Asian populations in England (Cruickshank et al 1985), and comparing native Jamaicans with whites in South Wales (Miall & Cochrane 1961) do not show this difference, and US studies which have standardised for social class have reduced or abolished 'racial' differences (Langford 1981). Social class remains a huge and neglected body of association and causation, still lacking a plausible explanation in biological terms. Low social class is a more powerful independent predictor of risk from ischaemic heart disease than blood cholesterol, smoking, or hypertension (Rose & Marmot 1981) and seems to be the most consistent factor underlying the large between-population differences found by Shaper et al (1981) in their study of coronary risk factors in British towns. This has now been confirmed by the studies of the national birth cohort, showing consistent, though smaller, social class differences in 36-year-old men (Wadsworth et al 1985). This is now the most promising, and most neglected, field of epidemiological enquiry into the causes of primary hypertension.

CONCLUSION

It seems best to admit that though stressful lives are unpleasant and best avoided (even if we cannot define them), and present levels of sodium intake are almost certainly not beneficial (even if we cannot define an intake threshold below which to aim), neither of these yet provide a basis for convincing plans for specific prevention that can be applied to the whole population in Britain. There is a better case for campaigns to reduce dietary sodium in countries like Japan and Portugal, with much higher average intakes.

However, taking a broader perspective and tackling all main risks for coronary heart disease and stroke, there is convincing evidence for the following public and personal policies:

> Stop cigarette smoking.
> Tackle obesity in young adults.
> Ask about alcohol intake as a routine and make the 4–8 units a day threshold for negative cardiovascular effects known to the public.
> Eat less animal fat, including eggs and milk products.
> Eat more cereals, fruit, vegetables, and fish.
> Take regular exercise.

If these steps were taken by most people, the entire distribution of blood pressure could well shift 10 mmHg or more to the right, and as Rose (1981) first pointed out, this could have a greater effect than any amount of individual antihypertensive treatment at the top end of the distribution.

REFERENCES

Arkwright P D, Beilin L J, Rouse I et al 1982 Effects of alcohol use and other aspects of lifestyle on blood pressure levels and prevalence of hypertension in a working population. Circulation 66:60

Bjorntorp P 1985 Obesity and the risk of cardiovascular disease. Annals of Clinical Research 17:3

Connor E B, Khaw K T 1985 Is hypertension more benign when associated with obesity? Circulation 72:53

Cooper R, Liu K, Trevisan M et al 1983 Urinary sodium excretion and blood pressure in children: absence of a reproducible association. Hypertension 5:135

Cruickshank J K, Jackson S H D, Beevers D G et al 1985 Similarity of blood pressure in Blacks, whites and Asians in England: the Birmingham factory study. Journal of Hypertension 3:365

Hamilton M, Pickering G W, Roberts J A F et al 1954 The aetiology of essential hypertension. I: The arterial pressure in the general population. Clinical Science 13:11

Hawthorne V M, Greaves D A, Beevers D G 1974 Blood pressure in a Scottish town. British Medical Journal iii:600

Haynes S G, Levine S, Scotch N et al 1978 The relationship of psychosocial factors to coronary heart disease in the Framingham study. I: Methods and risk factors. American Journal of Epidemiology 107:362

Haynes R B, Harper A C, Costley S R et al 1984 Failure of weight reduction to reduce mildly elevated blood pressure: a randomised trial. Journal of Hypertension 2:535

Henry J P 1980 Present concept of stress theory. In: Usdin E, Kvetnansky R, Kopin I J (eds) Catecholamines and stress. Elsevier, Oxford, p 557

Hofman A, Hazebroek A, Valkenburg H A 1983 A randomised trial of sodium intake and blood pressure in newborn infants. Journal of the American Medical Association 250:370

Kesteloot H, Geboers J 1982 Calcium and blood pressure. Lancet i:813

Langford H 1981 Is blood pressure different in black people? Postgraduate Medical Journal 57:749

Langford H G 1983 Electrolyte intake and excretion and its correlation with blood pressure: studies in children and adults. In: Gross F, Strasser T (eds) Mild hypertension: recent advances. Raven Press, New York

Miall W E, Cochrane A L 1961 The distribution of arterial pressure in Wales and Jamaica. Pathology and Microbiology 24:690

Petitti D B, Klatsky A L 1983 Malignant hypertension in women aged 15 to 44 years and its relation to cigarette smoking and oral contraceptives. American Heart Journal 52:297

Puska P, Iacono J M, Nissinen A et al 1983 Controlled randomised trial of the effect of dietary fat on blood pressure. Lancet i:1

Rose G A 1981 Strategies of prevention: lessons from cardiovascular disease. British Medical Journal 282:1847

Rose G, Marmot M G 1981 Social class and coronary heart disease. British Heart Journal 45:13

Rouse I L, Beilin L J 1984 Vegetarian diet and blood pressure. Journal of Hypertension 2:231

Samuelsson O, Wilhelmsen L, Elmfeldt D et al 1985 Predictors of cardiovascular morbidity in treated hypertension: results from the primary preventive trial in Goteborg, Sweden. Journal of Hypertension 3:167

Shaper A G, Pocock S J, Walker M et al 1981 British Regional Heart Study: cardiovascular risk factors in middle-aged men in 24 towns. British Medical Journal 283:179

Shekelle R B, Schoenberger J A, Stamler J 1976 Correlates of the JAS type A behaviour pattern score. Journal of Chronic Disease 29:381

Wadsworth M E J, Cripps H A, Midwinter R E et al 1985 Blood pressure in a national birth cohort at the age of 36 related to social and familial factors, smoking, and body mass. British Medical Journal 291:1534

Watt G C M, Foy C J W 1982 Dietary sodium and arterial pressure: problems of studies within a single population. Journal of Epidemiology and Community Health 36:197

Watt G C M, Foy C J W, Hart J T 1983 Comparison of blood pressure, sodium intake, and other variables in offspring with and without a family history of high blood pressure. Lancet i:1245

Watt G C M, Foy C J W, Hart J T et al 1985 Dietary sodium and arterial blood pressure: evidence against genetic susceptibility. British Medical Journal 291:1525

4

Iatrogenic hypertension

The commonest iatrogenic cause of apparent hypertension is to see it when it isn't there, by hasty diagnosis, poor conditions and technique of measurement, and poorly organised follow-up, as dealt with in Chapters 8, 9 and 10. The commonest iatrogenic causes of real hypertension or unexplained resistance to antihypertensive drugs are sympathomimetic amines, monoamine oxidase (MAO) inhibitors, carbenoxolone, non-steroidal anti-inflammatory drugs (NSAIDs) and the contraceptive pill.

SYMPATHOMIMETIC AMINES

These are contained in across-the-counter self-prescribed and doctor-prescribed cold remedies, appetite suppressants and CNS stimulants related to amphetamine. Illegally produced and procured amphetamine is another possibility in young patients with unexpectedly high pressures. Sympathomimetic amines usually cause psychiatric rather than cardiovascular symptoms, but forgotten use or unsuspected abuse of these drugs is an occasional cause of raised pressure, or of hypertension inexplicably resistant to treatment. Phenylephrine eye-drops used in newborn infants have been found to raise blood pressure by 25%, and a persistent systolic pressure of 130–160 mmHg was caused in one 7-week-old by 6-hourly eye drops containing 10% phenylephrine and 0.25% pseudoephedrine (Chaplin 1984).

These drugs tend to be overprescribed and all of them seem to create dependency in some people. Prescription of stimulant appetite suppressants can rarely be justified.

MONOAMINE OXIDASE INHIBITORS

Monoamine oxidase inhibitors are effective antidepressant drugs, useful because they act more quickly than tricyclic or quadricyclic antidepressants, do not cause the often troublesome anticholinergic side-effects of tricyclics, and are less effective suicidal agents. For all these reasons they remain useful drugs despite a bad reputation, earned during the early years when their interactions with amine-containing foods and drugs were not fully understood.

Patients on MAO inhibitors who are taking amines by self-medication or prescription, or in foods such as cheese, yeast extracts like Marmite, red wine, stout, or any smoked or traditionally preserved food that may contain putrefactive elements, are liable to acute hypertensive crises which may precipitate stroke. This is even more likely in patients who are already hypertensive, and MAO inhibitors should never be used for subjects whose blood pressure is already raised. When these drugs are used, these risks and their mechanism should be explained simply, backed up by written material. Medical records should be clearly marked to alert other health workers.

CARBENOXOLONE

Carbenoxolone is an effective treatment for gastric ulcer, somewhat less used since the advent of cimetidine. Like liquorice from which it is derived, it resembles deoxycorticosterone in its chemical structure and has mineralocorticoid activity. It causes water and sodium retention, and at daily doses of about 300 mg effects a rise of 15–30 mmHg systolic and 3–25 mmHg diastolic pressure (Nicholls & Espiner 1983).

NON-STEROIDAL ANTI-INFLAMMATORY DRUGS

Prostaglandin synthetase inhibitors such as indomethacin and its multitude of descendants cause sodium retention and antagonise the antihypertensive effects of beta-blockers and diuretics. It is still uncertain whether NSAIDs themselves cause a rise in pressure, or only antagonise the effects of antihypertensive medication (Watkins et al 1980), but both possibilities need to be kept in mind because NSAIDs are so commonly prescribed.

ORAL CONTRACEPTIVES

Because of the massive scale on which they are used and the early age at which they are applied, any contribution of oral contraceptives (OC) to cardiovascular risk is of enormous importance, most of all in primary care which is the only effective site for integrated control and monitoring. This is a subject on which all GPs should be well informed, and should formulate responsible practice policies.

The low universal rise

Figure 4.1 shows changes in systolic pressure after 2 years in 186 women aged 21–30 on combined oestrogen-progestogen OC compared with 60 controls (Weinberger & Weir 1983). There is a mean rise of nearly 8 mmHg in the women on OC compared with controls, and follow-up after another 3 years (5 years in all) showed a difference in the same direction of 12 mmHg systolic and 8 mmHg diastolic pressure.

This rise is not easily recognised in general practice, because OC

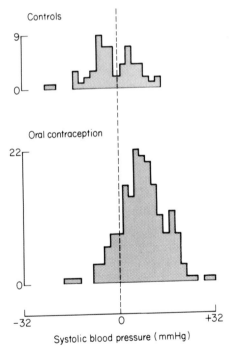

Fig. 4.1 Changes in systolic blood pressure after 2 years in women aged 21–30 years taking oestrogen–progestogen oral contraceptives (n = 186; mean = + 7.7 mmHg) and in controls (n = 60; mean = − 1.2 mmHg) (Weinberger & Weir 1983). (Reproduced with permission from: *Handbook of Hypertension* edited by J. I. S. Robertson, Elsevier, 1983).

is applied to a very young age-group in which even a rise of 10 or 20 mmHg of systolic pressure still remains well below the levels we have been taught to be alarmed at, and because if their pressures are monitored regularly every 3 months or so, as they should be, the initial apparent fall caused by habituation may exceed the underlying rise in true mean pressure. Most girls in their teens have systolic pressures around 100 mmHg, and most of us are not used to responding to changes from this very low starting point. Figure 4.2 demonstrates this.

This small rise seems to occur in nearly all women after about 6 months on OC. The huge Royal College of General Practitioners' controlled study of long-term risks showed a five-fold increase in

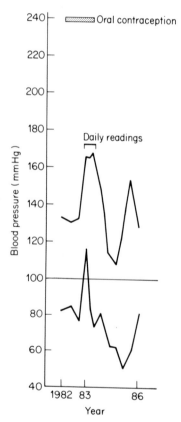

Fig. 4.2 Pressures recorded in a young woman (DT, born 29 May 1965) on oral contraceptives.

cardiovascular deaths in OC-users (25.8/100 000 woman-years) compared with non-users (5.5/100 000 woman-years), rising to 10-fold after 5 years. Most but certainly not all of this added risk is of thromboembolism, but there is also increased risk of subarachnoid haemorrhage and coronary disease, which may be hypertension-related. These data refer to the older OC formulations with 50 μ g oestrogen. With the 30 μ g and even lower preparations now in general use, risks are probably less, but they must still be taken seriously, and so far as possible reduced by regular monitoring verified by audit. It seems doubtful whether this is yet generally the case.

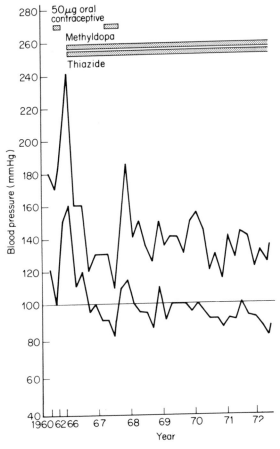

Fig. 4.3 Blood pressure record of female patient (MMJ, born 1 October 1927).

The high exceptional rise

Figure 4.3 shows pressures recorded for a Glyncorrwg woman on OC before the effect of OC on arterial pressure was known. These are frightening pressures, and fear is justified. In 1975 a case was reported of a 27-year-old woman, previously normotensive, who developed a systolic pressure of 180 mmHg on oestrogen-progestogen OC. Pressure fell to normal when OC was stopped, but after the next pregnancy OC was resumed, blood pressure rose to 250/160 mmHg, she developed malignant hypertension and died of irreversible renal failure (Zech et al 1975).

REFERENCES

Chaplin S 1984 Adverse reactions to sympathomimetics in cold remedies. Adverse Drug Reaction Bulletin no. 107, p 396
Nicholls M G, Espiner E A 1983 Liquorice, carbenoxolone and hypertension. In: Robertson J I S (ed) Handbook of hypertension. Elsevier Science Publishers, Oxford, p 189
Watkins J, Abbott E C, Hensby C N et al 1980 Attenuation of hypotensive effect of propranolol and thiazide diuretics by indomethacin. British Medical Journal 281:702
Weinberger M H, Weir R J 1983 Oral contraceptives and hypertension. In: Robertson J I S (ed) Handbook of hypertension. Elsevier Science Publishers, Oxford, p 196
Zech P, Rifle G, Lindner A et al 1975 Malignant hypertension with irreversible renal failure due to oral contraceptives. British Medical Journal iv:326

5

Natural history and complications

The natural history of high blood pressure falls naturally into two parts: its history as a risk factor, without local organ damage or symptoms; and its history as a disease, with organ damage, and sometimes with symptoms. This in turn may be subdivided into small artery disease, which is uniquely caused by severe hypertension, and large artery disease, in which hypertension is only one of several contributory causes. There will also be some discussion of unnatural history, that is, the extent to which organ damage can or cannot be avoided by reducing pressure.

CHANGES IN BLOOD PRESSURE OVER TIME

Changes with time are changes with both age and cumulative environmental effects. Figures 5.1 and 5.2 show trends in mean blood pressure in 1661 men and women randomly sampled from the general population of the Rhondda Fach and the Vale of Glamorgan, and followed up four times over the next 10 years (Miall & Chinn 1973). Obviously, most of the bundles of sticks show a rise with age, but not all of them, and steep rises and falls are shown from both high and low levels of initial pressure. None of these subjects was on antihypertensive medication.

NATURAL REGRESSION OF HIGH BLOOD PRESSURE?

Despite general tendencies for all blood pressures to rise with time and age in industrialised societies, and for high pressures to rise faster than low ones, these generalisations cannot be applied to individual patients. This is partly because arterial pressure is a relatively unstable variable, and one, two, or even three pressures recorded on separate days may not be truly representative of a patient's mean pressure over days or weeks. Blood pressure may also fall without treatment in subjects going into heart failure. But is it not also possible that in some people the hypertensive process

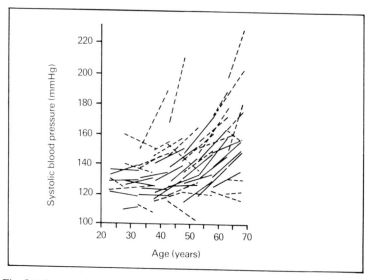

Fig. 5.1 Trends of mean systolic pressure for men followed up for 10 years, grouped according to systolic pressure and age at entry. Continuous lines = groups with 10 or more subjects; dashed lines = groups with less than 10 subjects (Miall & Chin 1973).

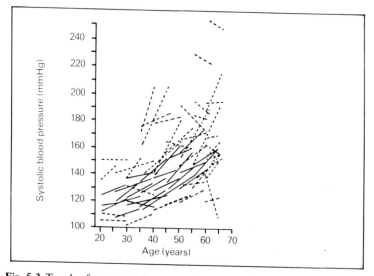

Fig. 5.2 Trends of mean systolic pressure for women followed up for 10 years, grouped according to systolic pressure and age at entry. Continuous lines = groups with 10 or more subjects; dashed lines = groups with less than 10 subjects (Miall & Chin 1973).

is transient rather than permanent, and that after a few months or years, even a well documented high pressure may undergo a sustained fall without treatment? This seems to have occurred in both the Australian (ANBPS; 1980) and the Medical Research Council (MRC; 1985) trials in many of the untreated or placebo-treated controls. In the ANBPS trial nearly 2000 untreated mild hypertensives were followed up. Mean pressure (three readings) fell from 158/102 mmHg at entry to 144/91 mmHg 3 years later; 9% rose by more than 10 mmHg, 22% fell by more than 10 mmHg, and 69% remained within 10 mmHg of their entry pressures. In the MRC trial, more than 7000 placebo-treated hypertensives were followed up, with mean entry pressures (four readings) of 158/96 mmHg. Over the next three years of follow-up 18% had diastolic pressures <90 mmHg at all anniversary visits.

Studying the behaviour of GPs in Scotland, Parkin et al 1979 found that over a third of all hypertensive patients' medication was started after a single reading, and there is no reason to think the results would have been different elsewhere in Britain. In the light of these Australian data, the misclassification and unnecessary treatment resulting from this slipshod policy are obvious.

However, if the original diagnosis of hypertension is supported by three or more readings a week or more apart, misclassification seems to be unusual. In preparing the second edition of this book, I was confident that I had in the Glyncorrwg population several examples of people with originally high and sustained pressures who for one reason or another were not treated, whose pressures subsequently fell, and who lived happily ever after. A careful search through the records of all the apparent candidates revealed not a single valid example of this process; those whose blood pressures fell in subsequent years all either had erratic readings when first detected, or were later found to have either heart failure or serious underlying disease causing the fall in pressure.

In general, blood pressures rise with time, and rise fastest in those with the highest pressures. High blood pressure is in most cases self-accelerating unless and until it is controlled by medical intervention of some kind, but rapid acceleration hardly ever occurs from diastolic pressures below 90 mmHg over 10 years of follow-up (Miall & Chinn 1974).

MALIGNANT HYPERTENSION

At any age, people with diastolic pressures sustained over

120 mmHg are at risk of malignant hypertension, in which pressure accelerates very fast, with a destructive effect on arteriolar networks in the brain, retina and kidney which may become irreversible even before alerting symptoms occur.

The classical criteria for diagnosis of malignant hypertension are not only very high pressure, but also the presence of neuroretinopathy; fluffy white patches usually close to the disc, often radiating fanwise toward the macula, usually accompanied by retinal haemorrhages, often with papilloedema, and almost always with proteinuria. Without papilloedema, purists have insisted that this is only 'accelerated hypertension'. In fact the clinical features and survival rate of accelerated hypertension and malignant hypertension are the same (Ahmed et al 1986), and the distinction is not useful.

Nearly all forms of retinal damage are commoner in people with high blood pressure, not only retinal haemorrhage, but retinal detachment and central retinal arterial occlusion. Again the association is causal and reversible, but fluffy white exudates (actually, oedema of the retinal capillary bed) and papilloedema are unique to the malignant phase, evidence of the small artery disease characteristic of rapidly accelerating severe hypertension, with arteriolar necrosis and multiple small infarcts.

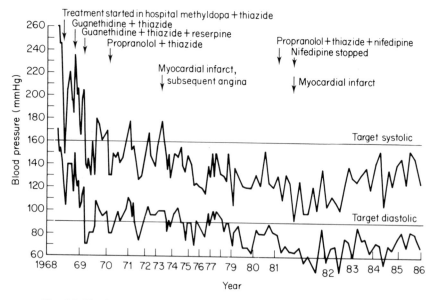

Fig. 5.3 Blood pressure record of male patient CD over 17 years' treatment, aged 43 in 1968

Similar arteriolar necrosis occurs in the brain, sometimes causing hypertensive encephalopathy with headache, transient symptoms and signs of brain injury due to multiple small infarcts, other times leading to frank haemorrhage and permanent brain damage or death.

Renal damage is invariable, but often asymptomatic, and is caused by the same process of fibrinoid necrosis of arterioles with multiple small infarcts. There is proteinuria, and a raised serum urea and creatinine. Even without symptoms, renal damage may become progressive and irreversible if pressure control is delayed too long.

Malignant hypertension in young women seems usually to be associated with underlying causal renal disease, cigarette smoking, oral contraception, or all three (Petitti et al 1983).

The Glyncorrwg man whose blood pressure record over 17 years

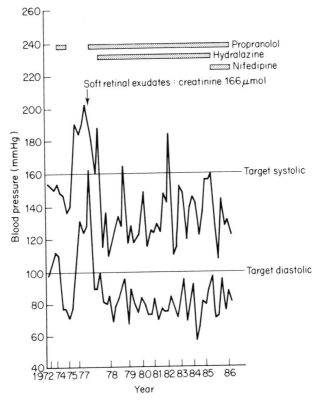

Fig. 5.4 Blood pressure record of male patient DN, aged 46 in 1972.

is shown in Figure 5.3 was lucky. Aged 43 when his blood pressure was first recorded at screening, he was found to have a diastolic pressure of 170 mmHg and a serum urea of 13 mmol(80 mg)/dl. He had no symptoms whatever, and no evidence of retinopathy. His impaired kidney function quickly returned to normal after pressure control was achieved.

Figure 5.4 shows pressures recorded for a man from an adjoining village who was not included in the 1968 screen. Because of poor practice organisation, several measurements of very high pressures were recorded before his retinopathy was recognised and pressure was controlled.

Neither of these men had disabling symptoms; both were on the brink of brain destruction or irreversible kidney failure. There is no way of looking for these uncommon cases of extremely dangerous hypertension, which does not entail measurement of all blood pressures in the whole adult population; in other words, some form of screening. Are these cases really so uncommon? In populations of 1700–2000 I have seen 4 in 30 years. It depends what you mean by 'common'; as common lives acquire more real and less rhetorical value, perhaps the word should be redefined.

THE SYMPTOMS OF HYPERTENSION

There are two sets of hypertensive symptoms; symptoms *of* hypertension, and symptoms *with* hypertension.

At diastolic pressures of 130 mmHg or more, headaches are commoner in hypertensives than in normotensive controls (Al Badran et al 1970), but below this level there is no difference with the prevalence of headache in random samples of the general population (Waters 1971). Robinson (1969) studied the relation of alleged classical hypertensive symptoms (headache, dizziness, breathlessness, fatigue, palpitations, insomnia, anxiety, and depression) to the level of blood pressure, and to the decisions of patients to consult a doctor and of doctors (in the 1960s) to measure their blood pressure. The only symptom showing any significant association with pressure was breathlessness, and this is more likely to have been causally associated with obesity.

In the early 1950s, when tuberculosis was still common, the commonest indication for requesting a chest X-ray was not chronic cough, night sweats, weight loss, or haemoptysis, but simply the absence of a previous chest X-ray during the last 10 years; tuberculosis had to be actively sought everywhere, if it was to be fully ascertained before it caused irreversible damage. The same applies to measurement of blood pressure today. For too many patients, the first symptom of high blood pressure is stroke, ventricular failure, retinal artery occlusion, or myocardial infarction.

STROKE: WHAT CAN BE ACHIEVED BY ANTIHYPERTENSIVE TREATMENT?

All causes of brain infarction are very much commoner in hypertensives. There is a closer association with haemorrhage than with thrombosis or embolism, but all of these outcomes are closely associated with arterial pressure. Even more important, they are reversibly associated with pressure; if pressure is reduced, so is the risk.

In the social conditions of fully industrialised societies, about 15% of all strokes might be prevented by control of high blood pressure above a threshold of 170/100 mmHg. This is much less than the reduction by half which many of us assumed as a result of the Veterans Administration studies, for the simple reason that this and other hospital studies dealt with much sicker populations than those observed by GPs from population screening, and also because many strokes still occur at much lower levels of pressure.

Data from the Framingham study show that the proportion of all stroke events occurring at entry pressures equal to or higher than this threshold is never more than 39% (men 55–64 years), and is usually much less. The 15% estimate is obtained by applying a 45% reduction in strokes to this group, which is the average result in all the controlled trials at that level, plus the results of the MRC trial in the next lower diastolic range.

Attempts to control hypertension by screening whole populations and then offering personal treatment have given results consistent with this reasoning. The Busselton project in Australia (Cullen et al 1979) used a diastolic threshold of 100 mmHg, and participating GPs achieved adequate diastolic control in 68% of hypertensives so defined. Male stroke deaths fell from 28 in 1967–1972 (before the project) to 10 in 1973–1977, but for women there were 25 stroke deaths in both periods, and a quarter of the fatal strokes occurred in people below this diastolic threshold. In the North Karelia project in Finland (Tuomilento et al 1985) treatment and control of hypertension, though better than in a reference area outside the project, have not been good enough for reliable conclusions to be drawn.

Mechanisms of stroke

The mechanisms of stroke are:

> Ruptures of large berry aneurysms, usually resulting in subarachnoid haemorrhage;
>
> Ruptures of Charcot-Bouchard microaneurysms, usually resulting in intracerebral haemorrhage;
>
> Emboli of mural thrombi from atherosclerotic carotid arteries, often preceded by warning transient ischaemic attacks (TIAs). Emboli may also come from the heart after myocardial infarction, or (and commonly) after weeks or months of heart failure, and especially with rheumatic valvular disease. All of these (including valvular disease) are commonly associated with hypertension;
>
> Intracerebral infarcts, usually capsular or cerebellar, often with histological evidence of fibrinoid necrosis despite absence of other features of malignant hypertension during life. Preceding pressures have usually been very high.

Stroke risk is a direct and immediate function of blood pressure; unlike coronary disease, it is little affected by serum cholesterol level or smoking, though there is a larger association with obesity, diabetes, and high alcohol intake. However, there are major determinants of stroke other than blood pressure which must account for the steep decline in stroke, mainly in haemorrhagic stroke (Yates 1964), observed in all countries for at least the last 30 years (Charlton & Velez 1986). These other determinants seem to be related to social class; there has been a widening gap between upper and lower social classes in Britain in every decennial occupational mortality report since 1950. Analysing the similar fall in stroke mortality in New Zealand since 1950, Bonita and Beaglehole (1986) estimated that only 10% of the fall could be accounted for by antihypertensive treatment.

LARGE ARTERY KIDNEY DAMAGE

Kidney damage in hypertension is seen in three circumstances. Firstly, it may itself cause hypertension. Secondly, it may be caused by occlusion of atherosclerotic renal arteries, or by fibrinoid necrosis of the renal arterioles in malignant hypertension. Finally, though present, kidney damage may have little to do with hypertension, as either cause or effect. It is a good rule that, except in the malignant phase, uncomplicated hypertension is never itself the principal cause of renal failure; seriously impaired kidney function should never be attributed to hypertension alone. It is also a good rule that in all states of impaired renal function, however caused, good control or even moderately raised pressure can help to preserve renal function and delay end-stage failure. This is particularly important in diabetics.

HEART FAILURE

Like stroke and retinal damage, heart failure can be caused by high arterial pressure, and prevented by its control. Unlike them, it is often ignored or misdiagnosed. It is still necessary to teach many trainees that chronic cough may be the main presenting symptom of heart failure. Hypertensive heart failure is easy enough to recognise in the form of acute left ventricular failure, with paroxysmal nocturnal dyspnoea, wheezing, triple rhythm, crackles all over the lungs and a high blood pressure. It is not so easy to recognise in the form of untreated hypertension over many years, followed by 'normal' blood pressure as the left ventricle fails. These are the women with 'ischaemic heart failure', so-called because they are seen in a hospital without past evidence from their GP records.

RUPTURED AORTA

Ruptured aorta is a fairly common cause of sudden or rapid death (3 in 25 years in a population of roughly 2000), usually in long-standing severe hypertension. Abdominal aneurysms sometimes give warning symptoms and may be suspected clinically and confirmed radiologically by their calcified outline, as atheroma is always severe. Above a critical diameter of 6 cm, half of them rupture within a year; below this diameter, about one-fifth.

ANGINA AND CLAUDICATION

In unscreened populations, angina and claudication are common presenting symptoms of long-standing hypertension. Because high arterial pressure speeds the deposition of atheroma in large and medium arteries, angina and claudication tend to occur sooner in hypertensives than in normotensives, but this also depends on serum cholesterol levels and smoking. Both symptoms usually improve after control of pressure.

CORONARY THROMBOSIS AND SUDDEN DEATH

Before the advent of tolerable and effective antihypertensive drugs in the early 1960s, heart failure and stroke were the principal outcomes of hypertension seen at post-mortem. Now that these are preventable, myocardial infarction has replaced them as the most frequent outcome of treated hypertension.

Hypertension promotes coronary disease chiefly by accelerating atheroma, but a precondition for this seems to be a serum total cholesterol above a threshold of about 5 mmol (200 mg)/dl. In populations with average cholesterol levels below this threshold, in Japan and black Africa for example, coronary disease is rare, despite widespread severe hypertension and heavy smoking.

YOU HAVE TO DIE SOMEHOW

The lethal outcomes of hypertension are, with few exceptions, relatively quick and easy exits compared with other common causes of death, such as cancer, dementia, and Parkinson's disease. Figure 5.5 shows the course of ineffectively treated hypertension in a vigorous old lady who finally died quickly with a massive myocardial infarct. Her hypertension might have been better controlled with more ruthless opposition to her systematic non-compliance (mainly because of side-effects from medication), but at her age a better outcome would have been unlikely. Mortality data which confuse tragedies in middle age with natural termination in the elderly do not contribute to reasoned argument.

BURSTING EFFECTS AND BLOCKING EFFECTS

With the single exception of the US Hypertension Detection and Follow-up Program (HDFP), which had neither untreated nor placebo-treated controls, all controlled trials of antihypertensive treatment have shown a big reduction in stroke morbidity and mortality (generally around 45% in the high-risk subgroups selected for trials), heart failure, and ruptured aorta, but little or no effect on morbidity or mortality from coronary heart disease. Indeed, one of the biggest trials, the Multiple Risk Factor Intervention Trial (MRFIT), actually showed a significant increase in coronary events in subjects taking antihypertensive drugs.

This is a difficult conclusion for activist GPs to accept, and an even more difficult conclusion to pass on to their patients, most of whom probably believe that prevention of coronary disease, rather than stroke or heart failure, is the main aim of treatment. Coronary deaths are about three times as common as stroke deaths, and much more fashionable as a cause for concern.

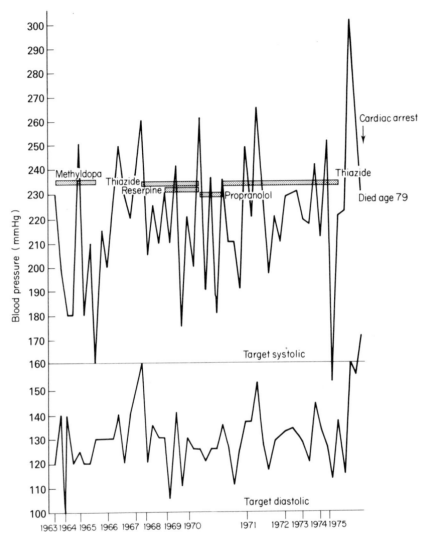

Fig. 5.5 Blood pressure record of female patient HD, aged 67 in 1963.

Figure 5.6 is a reminder of how effective treatment of severe hypertension can be in preventing stroke in these very high-risk patients, and how important it is to keep trying. In 162 hypertensive patients who had already survived one stroke, Figure 5.6 compares subsequent cardiovascular events in three groups: those

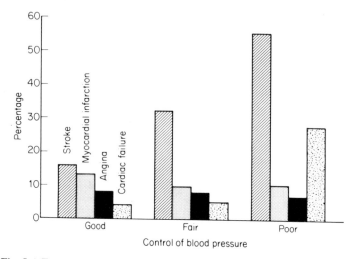

Fig. 5.6 Frequency of cardiovascular and cerebrovascular x disease in relation to control of blood pressure (Beevers et al 1973). (Reproduced with permission from *The Lancet*).

with good control (mean diastolic pressure <100 mmHg), fair control (mean diastolic pressure 100–109 mmHg), and poor control (mean diastolic pressure >110 mmHg). The patients were followed up for an average of 4 years.

There is a hugely obvious difference in the amount of stroke and heart failure according to quality of control, but very little (and that in the wrong direction) for myocardial infarction.

The bursting effects of hypertension (brain haemorrhages and capsular infarcts, fibrinoid arteriolar necrosis in the brain, retina and kidney, ruptured aorta, and overloaded left ventricle) are caused by hypertension alone, and are preventable by assiduous control of blood pressure. The blocking effects of hypertension (angina, claudication and myocardial infarction) are accelerated by hypertension, but are causally related more closely to smoking and serum cholesterol levels. They are preventable and to a considerable extent reversible by attention to these two risk factor, but not by control of arterial pressure.

These conclusions are no longer in reasonable doubt, but defeatism is no more justified now than it was when mass control of hypertension was first tackled, with the crude ideas and high hopes then current. How this more complex and sophisticated evidence might be incorporated in an effective programme of coronary as well as stroke and heart failure prevention is the subject of Chapter 6.

OUTCOME OF HYPERTENSION IN DEVELOPING COUNTRIES

Despite the low pressures found in some hunter–gatherer populations, high blood pressure in the Third World is generally at least as common in urbanised populations as in industrialised countries, in many cases more so. Because serum total cholesterol levels in the Third World (even in cities) are generally low, with even the top of the distribution below 5 mmol(200 mg)/dl, coronary heart disease remains rare despite both high blood pressure and very heavy smoking. Coronary disease has become a disease of the poor in developed countries, but remains a disease of the rich in poor countries. The principal outcomes of high blood pressure in poor countries are renal and heart failure and (above all) stroke.

For example, in Beijing, capital of China, accurate age-specific mortality rates for stroke and coronary heart disease, and for the prevalence of risk factors in the general population, are now available (Yingkai 1983). Men aged 55 had a stroke mortality of 633 and women a rate of 428 per 100 000, compared with coronary mortality rates of 129 and 51 per 100 000 respectively; five times as many fatal strokes as coronary deaths in men, and eight times as many in women. Mean cholesterol levels at age 55 were about 4.6 mmol (175 mg)/dl in both sexes, and 67% of men and 16% of women smoked.

If figures like these are characteristic of most populations in black Africa, South America, Asia, and the Middle East, or at least more characteristic than the population in Framingham and other sources of good epidemiological data in the industrialised world, hypertension control is more urgent, and likely to be more immediately cost-effective, in the Third World than in the First. As a longer-term strategy, and assuming that food supply and distribution improve, only control of smoking or adoption of Japanese or Mediterranean types of national diet can prevent a disastrous conjunction of coronary heart disease rates that are rising, and stroke rates that have not yet fallen.

There are powerful pressures on all developing countries to follow the same strategies for hypertension control as those which have evolved in the wealthiest and most technically advanced countries, above all the USA. Most of the basic research, pharmaceutical development and marketing comes directly or indirectly from the USA. America dominates the world medical literature with a truly imperial capacity to ignore every language but its own, while making knowledge of its own research literature the test of scientific respectability. WHO, and the Pan-American Health Organization which runs WHO work in South and Central America from Washington, encourage poor countries to apply the results of epidemiological studies in developed countries rather than develop their own research base. Conferences on hypertension as a public health problem are financed by multinational pharmaceutical companies chiefly interested in wider markets for new and expensive hypertensive drugs. Doctors whose living depends chiefly on personal care of a small minority of fee-payers are more interested in finding personal solutions for their hypertensive patients than in devising and implementing effective strategies for blood pressure control in the whole population. Not unnaturally, the ruling and senior administrative classes, whose own ways of life and therefore pathology imitate as much of *Dallas* as they can afford, see the development of excellent hospital-based specialist care as the first priority for their national health services. One or two rural and shantytown clinics are developed to a point where they can have a token role in undergraduate education and can be visited by foreign specialists, but primary care gets the rhetoric while hospitals get whatever cash is left after the guns have been paid for.

The control of high blood pressure is much more important in poor countries than in rich ones, for three reasons. Firstly, high blood pressure is more important as a single reversible risk, causing stroke, malignant hypertension, and renal failure in the urban poor on a far greater scale than in countries with fully developed economies and a less unequal distribution of wealth. In urban black South Africans, for example, hypertension is the main cause of premature non-violent death (Seftel et al 1980). The cost-effectiveness of screening for high blood pressure and giving energetic and sustained antihypertensive treatment to people with severe hypertension would be far higher in these countries than in the USA or Britain.

Secondly, the virtual absence of personal medical services leaves a clear field for development of primary prevention, with action to increase dietary potassium and reduce dietary sodium, to reduce alcohol consumption, to control obesity and discourage smoking. The strong collective tradition which is a precondition for survival in poor communities is in many ways a better substrate for health education than wealthier societies seeking only personal solutions by acquisition of medical care.

Thirdly, because in most cases diets are not yet atherogenic, poor countries still have the possibility of avoiding the 'western' pattern of pathology, and of following a new path entirely. Though this is a theoretical possibility, it has not so far been realised anywhere in practice. The USSR and East European republics are now in a phase of very rapid acceleration in coronary mortality in early middle age, and Cuba now has an almost completely 'western' pattern of mortality. Common to all these countries have been high cigarette and in some cases high alcohol consumption, followed by a weight-gaining and atherogenic diet as planned targets for a universal minimum diet have been achieved. Against a probably unchanged background distribution of blood pressure, hypertensives in these countries have moved from the poverty-pattern of early stroke, heart failure and malignant hypertension to the affluent pattern of early death from myocardial infarction.

This second edition was originally planned to contain a chapter on management of hypertension in poor countries. For 25 years I have lived and worked in a community which once produced the wealth now concentrated in the south-east of England. Our male unemployment rates in the Afan valley have not been less than 40% since 1982, families are being broken up while our children roam the world looking for work, whole streets are falling into ruin. In many ways the South Wales valleys can claim to be the Third World of British society, encountering the same attitudes of condescension and sentimental hand-wringing from central power. In the end I have not written such a chapter, because all effective solutions are national and local, and writing about other people's problems is an impertinence. Real rather than abstract medical science is culture-dependent. Progress in primary care depends on the most peripheral health workers gaining confidence in their own ability to solve problems using their own experience from their own research base, which can be based on simple systems of clinical audit based on random samples from registered populations.

That is not to say that lessons cannot be learned across national boundaries, particularly from South Africa and the USA, where hugely unequal distributions of wealth provide both appropriate populations, and sophisticated research teams able to study them. A few references are given (Dalal 1980; Sever et al 1980; Mugambi 1981; Pinkney-Atkinson et al 1981; Pobee 1981; Saunders et al 1982; Wu Yingkai et al 1982; Wyndham 1982; Isaacson 1983; Liu

Li-Sheng 1983; Seedat 1983; Wasir et al 1983); what are still almost entirely missing from the world literature, however, are realistic accounts from peripheral health workers of the work they are actually doing or trying to do, and the difficulties and opportunities they encounter, expressed both in anecdotal and simple statistical terms. Only these practical health workers are in a position to contribute to serious discussion of the most important problem now facing medical science; not how to know more to help a few people, but how to get what we already know implemented for everyone who needs it.

REFERENCES

Ahmed M E K, Walker J M, Beevers D G et al 1986 Lack of difference between malignant and accelerated hypertension. British Medical Journal 292:235
Al Badran R H, Weir R J, McGuiness J B 1970 Hypertension and headache. Scottish Medical Journal 15:48
Australian National Blood Pressure Study Management Committee 1980 The Australian therapeutic trial in mild hypertension. Lancet i:1261
Beevers D G, Hamilton M, Fairman M J et al 1973 Antihypertensive treatment and the course of established cerebral vascular disease. Lancet i:1407
Bonita R, Beaglehole R 1986 Does treatment of hypertension explain the decline in mortality from stroke? British Medical Journal 292:191
Charlton J R H, Velez R 1986 Some international comparisons of mortality amenable to medical intervention. British Medical Journal 292:295
Cullen K J, McCall M G, Stenhouse N S 1979 Changing mortality due to strokes in men following treatment of Busselton hypertensives 1966–77. International Journal of Epidemiology 8:213
Dalal P M 1980 Hypertension: a report on community survey for casual hypertension in 'old' Bombay. Sir Hurkisondas Nurrotumdas Hospital Medical Research Society, Bombay.
Isaacson C 1983 The pathology of hypertension in a tropical environment. Clinical Cardiology 6:195
Liu Li-Sheng 1983 Epidemiological report from China. In: Gross F, Strasser T (eds) Mild hypertension: recent advances. Raven Press, New York, p 19
Medical Research Council Working Party 1985 MRC trial of treatment of mild hypertension: principal results. British Medical Journal 291:97
Miall W E, Chinn S 1973 Blood pressure and ageing; results of a 15–17 year follow-up study in South Wales. Clinical Science and Molecular Medicine 45:23s
Miall W E, Chinn S 1974 Screening for hypertension: some epidemiological observations. British Medical Journal 3:595
Mugambi M 1981 Epidemiological report from East Africa. South African Medical Journal 59:55
Parkin D M, Kellett R J, Maclean D W et al 1979 The management of hypertension: a study of records in general practice. Journal of the Royal College of General Practitioners 29:590
Petitti D B, Klatsky A L 1983 Malignant hypertension in women aged 15 to 44 years and its relation to cigarette smoking and oral contraceptives. American Journal of Cardiology 52:297

Pinkney-Atkinson V J, Milne M E, Fee L E et al 1981 The role of the advanced clinical nurse in a hypertension clinic. South African Medical Journal 59:563

Pobee J O M 1981 Epidemiological report from West Africa. South African Medical Journal 59:33

Robinson J O 1969 Symptoms and the discovery of high blood pressure. Journal of Psychosomatic Research 13:157

Saunders L D, Irwig L M, Wilson T D 1982 Hypertension management and patient compliance at a Soweto polyclinic. South African Medical Journal 61:147

Seedat Y K 1983 Race, environment and blood pressure: the South African experience. Journal of Hypertension 1:7

Seftel H C, Johnson S, Muller E A 1980 Distribution and biosocial correlations of blood pressure levels in Johannesburg Blacks. South African Medical Journal 57:313

Sever P S, Gordon D, Peart W S et al 1980 Blood pressure and its correlates in urban and tribal Africa. Lancet ii:60

Tuomilehto J, Nissinen A, Wolf E et al 1985 Effectiveness of treatment with antihypertensive drugs and trends in mortality from stroke in the community. British Medical Journal 291:857

Wasir H S, Ganai A M, Nath L M 1983 An epidemiological study of hypertension in an Indian rural community. Indian Heart Journal 35:294

Waters W E 1971 Headache and blood pressure in the community. British Medical Journal i:142

Wu Yingkai, Lu Chang-ging et al 1982 Nationwide hypertension screening in China during 1979–80. Chinese Medical Journal 95:101

Wyndham C H 1982 Trends with time of cardiovascular mortality rates in the populations of the RSA for the period 1968–77. South African Medical Journal 61:987

Yates P O 1964 A change in the pattern of cerebrovascular disease. Lancet i:65

Yingkai W 1983 Report of WHO Sino-MONICA for 1983. Not published, available on application from WHO Europe

Tables 2–2 and 8–2 in The Framingham study: an epidemiological investigation of cardiovascular disease (Section 30) Some characteristics related to the incidence of cardiovascular disease and death; Framingham Study, 18-year follow-up. Department of Health Education & Welfare publication no. (NIH) 74–599, US Government Printing Office, Washington DC, 1974. I am grateful to my colleague Graham Watt for drawing my attention to this, and doing the calculations.

6

Thresholds for intervention and follow-up

Since below a diastolic pressure of 130 mmHg symptoms are no commoner in hypertensives than in the normotensive population unless organ damage has already occurred, definitions of hypertension cannot depend on a presented complaint. They must either be arbitrary and idiosyncratic, or based on evidence of their usefulness in saving life and preventing organ damage, balanced against evidence of costs, both in iatrogenic impairment and consumption of social resources.

In the past, criteria for diagnosis have differed from criteria for treatment. One American study of factors influencing the decision to treat or not treat for high blood pressure found that only 20% of the variance could be accounted for by generally accepted clinical variables such as systolic and diastolic pressure, fundus changes, electrocardiogram (ECG) and biochemical evidence (Gibson et al 1978). This does not mean the other 80% of these decisions were irrational, but it does show that many factors which are usually ignored enter into clinical decisions.

These factors include real or presumed patient expectation, workload, doctors' opinions about the capacity of individual patients to cope with treatment or benefit from it, priority given to other potentially conflicting clinical or social problems the patient may have, and economic incentives and disincentives for enlarging the scope of care. For the past ten years at least, medical consensus on thresholds for treatment has differed on the two sides of the Atlantic, apparently because of differences in care systems, rather than scientific evidence. In the USA, medical interventions generate fees; in Britain they generate taxes.

THE PIONEER STUDIES

Effective antihypertensive drugs first became available in the middle 1950s, and were in wide use by the early 1960s. Because all of them caused serious side-effects, their use in hitherto asymptomatic patients was difficult and generally limited to a small market. The first evidence that their use could result in a net saving of life came from small controlled studies of subjects referred to hospital specialists with severe and immediately dangerous hypertension, nearly all of them with evidence of organ damage. Studying men and women of mean age around 50 with diastolic pressures >150 mmHg, Leishman (1963) increased 2-year survival by two-thirds in 34 patients who were treated, compared with 42 who were not. Hamilton et al (1964) studied men and women under the age of 60 without symptoms, and with diastolic pressures sustained over 110 mmHg for 3 months. They were allocated alternately to treatment and no treatment. In the men, 10 who were treated had no complications, but of the 12 controls, 4 had strokes and 1 had other complications. In the women, control of blood pressure in the treated group was poor; they had 3 strokes and 2 other complications, compared with 3 strokes and 5 other complications, an insignificant difference. Comparing only the 16 women with adequate control, only one complication occurred in the adequately treated group, compared with 6 strokes and 6 other complications in the other 23.

THE VETERANS ADMINISTRATION STUDIES

The two US Veterans Administration trials, begun in 1964, confirmed the results of these pioneer studies, and after publication in 1967 and 1970 became the classical evidence on which virtually all treatment policies claimed to be based. Like the pioneer studies, they were based on hospital-referred populations, with much more organ damage and a far higher complication rate than one would expect from a population sample of the same age and pressure. Diastolic thresholds were established from inpatient readings over 3 days, confirmed by three further outpatient readings before treatment. The Veterans' study began on 523 men aged 30–73 (mean age 50 years), divided into two groups, the first in the diastolic range 115–119 mmHg (Veterans Administration 1967) and the second 90–114 mmHg (Veterans Administration 1970). Controlled study of the 125 men with higher pressures was stopped after 3 years, because there were 4 deaths and 19 major complications (including 3 strokes) in the untreated controls, compared with no deaths and 1 major complication (a stroke) in the treated cases.

Part II of the Veterans' study, on 380 men in the pressure range

90–114 mmHg, continued for a full 5 years. There were 19 cardio-vascular deaths and 37 non-fatal complications in the controls, compared with 8 deaths and 13 complications in the cases random-ised to treatment. Benefit from treatment was significant for those with organ damage or with entry diastolic pressures at or over 105 mmHg; for those in the diastolic range 90–104 mmHg and without organ damage, they were barely significant.

THE HDFP

Is medical opinion based on evidence, or evidence based on medical opinion?

Although in 1976 the only available controlled evidence of signifi-cant benefit from treatment of hypertension was based on hospital-referred cases and began at a diastolic threshold of 105 mmHg, 78% of doctors in New York State were already prescribing anti-hypertensive drugs for people in the general population in the diastolic range 90–100 mmHg, and by 1979 (when there was still no controlled evidence of benefit) this proportion had risen to 90% (Guttmacher et al 1981). By the time a large enough US trial could be set up either to challenge or legitimise this consensus, it was already considered unethical to withhold treatment from anyone with a diastolic pressure over 90 mmHg. So the trial which even-tually took place, the Hypertension Detection and Follow-up Program (HDFP; 1979), instead of comparing treated cases with randomised untreated controls, compared the mortality results of a structured system of free treatment and active recall by specially trained nurse practitioners, with the results of the ordinary US medical market, assuming that this purpose-built structured care would be more rigorous than marketed care, particularly for mild hypertension. However, it did draw its subject from random samples of local populations rather than hospital-referred cases.

After 5 years, reductions of 26% for cardiovascular mortality and 13% for non-cardiovascular mortality were shown for the group receiving free, structured, active-recall care by nurses, compared with the group receiving traditional marketed care from doctors. Did American doctors therefore press their congressmen to legislate for a free primary care national health service staffed by nurse prac-titioners? They did not. The HDFP was used not to answer the question most appropriate to its design (which of these two kinds of health service works best?), but to reinforce what doctors were already doing. The results of the HDFP trial were published towards the end of 1979, just before the first edition of this book went to press. They could therefore not be taken into account, but even if they had been available they would not have altered its conclusion that mass pharmaceutical intervention in the diastolic range 90–104 mmHg is not justified by convincing evidence.

THE AUSTRALIAN TRIAL

The next important controlled evidence came from the Management Committee of the Australian National Blood Pressure Study (ANBPS), published in 1980. With much arm-twisting, of which I had personal experience, it was the basis for international guidelines endorsed unanimously by a World Health Organization (WHO) conference at Burgenstock in 1982.

The ANBPS followed men and women aged 30–69 with diastolic pressures 95–109 mmHg at entry for 4 years. They were volunteers from the general population, so instead of over-representing high morbidity, as all the hospital-based studies certainly did, the ANBPS was probably selective for hypertensives with least organ damage and lowest risk. It allocated subjects randomly to treatment or no treatment (there was no placebo group) so side-effects could not be measured. The study was relatively small, and was wound up as soon as differences between treated and control subjects reached the lower limits of significance.

An important finding was that the risk of complications in treated subjects was proportionate to achieved pressures rather than entry pressures, and this was subsequently confirmed in other trials, including analyses of the Veterans' studies. This showed that quality of care was all-important in achieving results.

As before, there was a large reduction in strokes, but a barely significant fall in coronary heart disease. The actual numbers of deaths in the two groups were 5 in the treated subjects and 11 in the controls; 2000 patient-years of treatment for each life saved.

THE COST-BENEFIT EQUATION

So low a yield for so great an effort must raise the question whether net gains exceeded net losses.

All treatments (even without medication) incur costs, in labour diverted from other possibly more useful tasks, and in iatrogenic impairments. We must recognise that ever since survival to old age became commonplace (a recent development even in the industrialised world) medical interventions can at best have had only marginal effects on mortality. Small iatrogenic impairments on a sufficiently large scale can therefore outweigh any advantages of medical intervention, and the scale of both actual and potential antihypertensive medication is enormous. Treatment of all blood pressures sustained over diastolic 90 mmHg includes about 15% of the adult population, and 30% of some urban ghetto areas.

As we saw in the last chapter, the MRFIT trial suggested that just such an effect may in fact have been operating to promote sudden heart death in hypertensives treated with thiazide diuretics and beta-blockers, by reducing plasma potassium and increasing total cholesterol levels. The effects of antihypertensive drugs on other risk factors must now be regarded as equally important as their efficacy in reducing blood pressure, and in mild hypertension, even more important.

THE PRE-MRC CONSENSUS

Despite its almost unmeasurably low yield, the ANBPS was hailed as validation of diastolic 95 mmHg as a threshold for treatment by WHO, and seemed to be viewed as a reasonable compromise between the US policy of zapping every pressure over 90 mmHg, and the British policy of waiting and seeing what the much larger and more tightly designed MRC trial would show. Certainly in the USA, and probably in Australia, treatment with antihypertensive drugs became the normal response of most doctors to all diastolic pressures sustained at or over 90 mmHg (phase V) through two or three readings. British doctors seem generally to have settled for a diastolic threshold of 100 mmHg, while awaiting a final verdict from the results of the MRC trial.

THE MRC TRIAL

The MRC trial (1985) was on a huge scale, with more than 17 000 subjects and 85 000 patient-years of observation, compared with 11 000 subjects and 55 000 patient-years in the HDFP. It had a single-blind randomised placebo-controlled design, and is likely to be the last trial of this size without actively treated controls. Using bendrofluazide and propranolol as its principal drugs for screened men and women aged 35–64 in the diastolic range 90–109 mmHg, it sought to answer two main questions: does treatment for this group reduce strokes or coronary events? And if so, what are the costs of these reductions in terms of iatrogenic impairment and medical, nursing and administrative labour?

Treatment reduced the number of strokes by 45%, agreeing well with all the earlier trials. However, strokes in this age group are rare, even in mild-to-moderate hypertensives, and it took 850 patient-years of treatment to prevent each one. An average GP list of about 2000 subjects of all ages will contain around 100 patients in this age and pressure group, so each GP might expect to prevent about one stroke every 8.5 years by finding and treating all of them.

Treatment had no effect on coronary events, and worse still, had no effect on all-cause mortality for both sexes combined, even if strokes are included. This was because the small reduction in cardiovascular deaths in men was counterbalanced by an increase in non-cardiovascular deaths in women, chiefly from cancer.

These results are based only on a 5-year follow-up, and it is probable though not certain that some benefits have yet to appear. Figure 6.1 shows the difference between treated and untreated subjects grew steadily through the 5 years of the Veteran Administration II trial; clearly it is reasonable to believe that benefits are greater, the longer control is maintained.

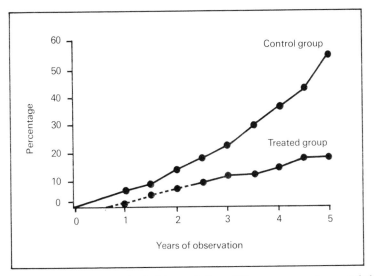

Fig. 6.1 Estimated cumulative incidence of all morbid events over a 5-year period for treated and control groups in Part II of the Veterans' Study. Life-table method (Veterans Administration 1970).

Control of mild-to-moderate hypertension in middle age will probably prevent a good deal of heart failure in the elderly, a lot more strokes, and conceivably some multi-infarct dementia. If we are lucky, it may prevent some coronary disease; atheroma certainly cannot be reversed quickly, but very prolonged treatment may be more effective.

DIFFERENCES BETWEEN THE TRIALS

How can we account for the differences between the MRC trial, which had no effect on coronary disease, and the ANBPS and HDFP, which had apparently positive results for coronary disease? The ANBPS was a relatively small trial (about 13 000 patient-years of observation) and was wound up on ethical grounds as soon as marginal levels of significance were reached for all terminations, both strokes and coronary events. Set against the sixfold greater size of the MRC trial, with at least as good a design and quality control, the simplest explanation is probably correct; the MRC and the ANBPS results approximate to the same truth, but the MRC comes closer because of its larger scale.

The HDFP was much bigger than the ANBPS and cannot be criticised for insufficient numbers. Interpretation is difficult because of the indirect design discussed above, with no untreated controls. Unlike the MRC trial, for which no subset results are yet available, HDFP results were given for three strata of blood pressure at entry: diastolic ranges 90–104 (Stratum I), 105–114 (Stratum II), and >115 mmHg (Stratum III), with 72% of subjects in Stratum I. In all strata there was a significant reduction in strokes and stroke mortality for patients receiving free structured care, compared with controls receiving marketed care, a result in line with other studies. Unlike them, however, there was also a 26% reduction in deaths from myocardial infarction, entirely restricted to Stratum I (diastolic 90–104 mmHg), and greatest in black women, followed by black men, and then by white men; there was no difference for white women. This suggests that gains from free structured care were greatest for the previously most disadvantaged groups, a theory reinforced by another remarkable, unexpected, and still unexplained finding in the HDFP; there was also a 13% reduction in non-cardiovascular mortality. Finally, 25% of Stratum I subjects were already on antihypertensive medication when they were screened, and the original pressures before treatment were not available; this group is therefore contaminated by an unknown but possibly considerable number of more severe hypertensives poorly controlled at entry.

SOCIAL COMPOSITION OF THE TRIALS

An outstanding and somewhat neglected difference between the MRC and ANBPS studies on the one hand, and the HDFP on the other, was their different social composition. The MRC was recruited from volunteer group practices with 10 000 or more patients. Its authors admit, and participating GPs readily confirm, that the participating practices were heavily biased toward comfortable middling town and suburban practice, areas with generally low morbidity and certainly not of the same social character as Glasgow, Liverpool, Belfast and the South Wales valleys, the really bad areas for both stroke and coronary mortality in Britain. The ANBPS was a patient volunteer study which seems to have attracted an unusually healthy population of probably above-average social class. In contrast to both of these, the HDFP drew on generally more sick, more urban, more black, more industrial, and more disadvantaged populations; Tyroler (1983) has written interestingly on this. Of male subjects 30% were black, compared with an expected value of about 10% for the general US population. All-causes mortality and stroke mortality in Stratum I of the HDFP free structured care group were each nearly three times higher than in the placebo group of the MRC trial, and coronary mortality was over twice as high. Primary care teams working in high mortality, high morbidity, and high unemployment areas of Britain may well feel greater affinity with the HDFP populations than the tweedy tendencies of the MRC trial. Perhaps treatment works better in neglected populations; if so, the lesson of the HDFP is that treatment should be structured and free, rather than entrepreneurial. This still does not help us define an effective threshold.

THE MRC TORPEDO

The fact remains that the MRC trial results have finally torpedoed any rational argument for antihypertensive medication in the diastolic range 90–110 mmHg, except where there is either positive evidence of organ damage, or exceptional risk of such damage, as in diabetics or those with a family history of stroke. A detailed analysis of the cost-effectiveness of treatment in the MRC trial range by Milner and Johnson (1985) supports this conclusion. No doubt it will remain unacceptable for a long time wherever medical intervention is buoyed up by fees, but eventually the ship will sink. In fact, if we look at the absolute rather than relative gains of the ANBPS, there was a large hole in it already.

In the NHS we have a more subtle problem. Having begun to mobilise primary care for a mass attack on hypertension, what are we to do with our army; demobilise and give up the war against arterial disease, or find a more effective way to fight? A limited retreat of some kind seems inevitable. And what policy are we to follow for patients already controlled on the old diastolic 100 consensus?

IS TREATMENT OF MILD HYPERTENSION WORTHWHILE?

It cannot be right to put 170 people in the diastolic range 90–109 mmHg on continuous antihypertensive medication and regular monitoring for 5 years, in order that one of them should avoid a stroke. The proportion of hypertensives for whom anti-hypertensive medication can now be justified is much smaller (about 4–10% of most British populations) than most of us once thought and hoped. Can the contribution of personal clinical care therefore be ignored in terms of public health strategy? In a well argued paper, Geoffrey Rose (1981) approaches this conclusion, which within the limits of our present NHS structure is probably justified.

The argument is wrong on two counts. First, 4–10% of the population is not a small number. Judging from the way we deal with diabetes, affecting only 2% of the population, it is a much larger number than we can cope with without some reorganisation of the health service, and epidemiologists and community physicians cannot simply turn their backs on the problem.

It is wrong also for a more fundamental reason. Even the most severe hypertension is usually asymptomatic at least until there is organ damage, and often remains so until (for example) renal, retinal, or brain damage become irreversible. However high the threshold is set, the only way to identify all the people who need antihypertensive medication is to screen everyone between the ages of 30 and 65 at least once every 5 years; but if such screening is carried out, it will detect much greater numbers of people below threshold, but at high relative risk. Are these people to be ignored, or are we going to do something positive to help them?

This is the central paradox of all strategies for hypertension control; detection and effective treatment of a few requires organised contact with everyone. Surely such organised mass contact with health workers, potentially motivated for prevention by their own experience of unprevented cardiovascular disease and skilled in personal care, should be maximally used?

The answer is to recognise that attempts to reduce blood pressure in isolation from control of other risk factors is futile. The only effective strategy is to accept hypertension as one of several risks, and the search for it as only one of several possible entry points to a final common pathway — reduction of premature coronary and stroke mortality by control of multiple risk factors in the whole population. Because in the British NHS the whole population is registered with GP's responsibility to all their patients means responsibility to all the people. Search for hypertension is a good entry point to this much larger task, because for historical reasons this is what most interested GPs have wanted to do, but the same point would eventually be reached by comprehensive search for any other risk factor; diabetes, obesity, smoking, airways obstruction, alcohol or hyperlipidaemia.

CONCLUSION: A THRESHOLD FOR MANDATORY TREATMENT

In the endless discussions about who should or should not be treated with antihypertensive drugs at the broad base of the hypertensive pyramid, we are in danger of losing sight of the apex of severe, imminently dangerous hypertension, in which the need for effective treatment is beyond doubt. Though the results of the MRC trial suggest that this threshold might lie around 195/110 mmHg (phase V), a look at the Framingham data shown in Figure 6.2 suggests a more reasonable division around 175/105 mmHg, the point at which the really steep rise in risk begins. This is in fact the threshold implied by the Veterans Administration studies.

On the best controlled evidence we are ever likely to have, antihypertensive medication is mandatory for blood pressure sustained at or over 175/105 mmHg, using either a systolic or diastolic value, whichever is the higher. Below this threshold, decisions to treat with antihypertensive drugs should be based on a family history of stroke or ruptured aorta, rapid progression of pressure, evidence of organ damage, complicating disease (mainly

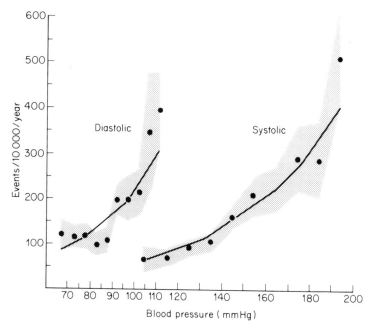

Fig. 6.2 Annual incidence of cardiovascular events at Framingham over 18 years of follow-up, by level of blood pressure in all ages, and with mean of male and female rates. Shaded areas indicate 95% confidence limits of individual data points, based on the assumption that the numbers of events behave as Poisson variables. (Anderson 1978). (Reproduced with permission from *The Lancet*).

diabetes), onset under the age of 40, or interacting risk factors which are discussed in Chapter 7. The largely negative results of the MRC trial should not be misused to endorse passivity in tackling necessary and effective work which is still less than half done.

REFERENCES

Anderson T W 1978 Re-examination of some of the Framingham blood pressure data. Lancet ii:1139

Gibson E S, Sackett D L, Haynes R B et al 1978 Clinical determinants of the decision to treat primary hypertension. In: Abstracts of the 18th conference on cardiovascular disease epidemiology, CVD Epidemiology Newsletter no. 25. American Heart Association, Dallas

Guttmacher S, Teitelman M, Chapin G et al 1981 Ethics and preventive medicine: the case of borderline hypertension. In: Hastings Center Report,

February. This paper cites evidence from the New York Heart Association and from the New York State Journal of Medicine 1979; 79:754

Hamilton M, Thompson E N, Wisniewski T K M 1964 The role of blood pressure control in preventing complications of hypertension. Lancet i:235

Hypertension Detection and Follow-up Program Cooperative Group 1979 Five-year findings of the HDFP, I and II. Journal of the American Medical Association 242:2562

Leishman A W D 1963 Merits of reducing high blood pressure. Lancet i:1284

Management Committee, Australian National Blood Pressure Study 1980 The Australian therapeutic trial in mild hypertension. Lancet i:121

Medical Research Council Working Party 1985 MRC trial of treatment of mild hypertension: principal results. British Medical Journal 291:97

Milner P C, Johnson I S 1985 Treating mild hypertension. Lancet ii:1364

Rose G A 1981 Strategies of prevention: lessons from cardiovascular disease. British Medical Journal 282:1847

Tyroler H A 1983 Race, education, and 5-year mortality in HDFP Stratum I referred-care males. In: Gross F, Strasser T (eds) Mild hypertension: recent advances. Raven Press, New York, p 163

Veterans Administration Co-operative Study Group on Antihypertensive Agents 1967 Effects of treatment on morbidity in hypertension I: results in patients with diastolic blood pressures averaging 115 through 129 mmHg. Journal of the American Medical Association 202:116

Veterans Administration Co-operative Study Group on Antihypertensive Agents 1970 Effects of treatment on morbidity in hypertension II: results in patients with diastolic pressures averaging 90 through 114 mmHg. Journal of the American Medical Association 213:1143

World Health Organization/International Society of Hypertension Conference 1982 Memorandum on guidelines for the treatment of mild hypertension. WHO Cardiovascular Diseases Unit, Geneva

7

Hypertension as one of several risk factors

Control of severe hypertension can still to some useful extent be regarded as an isolated objective, because the disease has at least one outcome unique to itself, malignant hypertension. Even so, most of the effects of even severe hypertension overlap with more general causes of arterial disease and ischaemic organ damage. Policies for control of mild and moderate hypertension, on the other hand, become completely irrational unless they take full account of other risk factors for arterial disease. The implications of this are precise; instead of measuring, explaining, treating and monitoring blood pressure in about 7% of the total population, we need measurement, explanation, treatment and monitoring of all major risk factors in at least twice that number; we need to know four times as much about twice as many people.

PANDORA'S BOX

There is worse to come. The problem may appear just conceivably manageable if we limit responsibility to the 15% or so of the population with blood pressures sustained over 150/90 mmHg; but there are equally compelling theoretical arguments for defining it by the 16% with life-shortening obesity (body mass index >30), the 35% who smoke, or the 15% with serum cholesterol >6.5 mmol (250 mg)/dl. Even more theoretically convincing are the arguments for tackling all those who have two or more major risks, which means over 80% of the adult population under retirement age.

In real life, risk factors cannot be isolated. High blood pressure, smoking, obesity, high blood cholesterol and diabetes do not exist on their own as diseases; they are distortions of normal physiology usually occurring more than one at a time.

The separate and variously combined effects of the three biggest treatable risk factors have been studied in several large surveys in the USA, the results of which were combined in the Pooling Project (Stamler & Epstein 1972). Defining the risk factors as:

1. total blood cholesterol >6.5 mmol (250 mg)/dl,
2. diastolic blood pressure >90 mmHg, and
3. any current use of cigarettes,

the project found an exponential rise in the risk of coronary events for men with all three risk factors, compared with those with any two, any one, or none at all, as shown in Figure 7.1. Taking the numbers of men at risk in the bottom line of Figure 7.1, Figure 7.2 shows the proportions of US white men aged 30–59 years with these risk combinations (British figures are even worse). Of the 7342 in this study, 38% had either any two or all three risk factors present as defined. These accounted for 58% of first coronary events during 10 years of follow-up, 62% of all sudden deaths, and 55% of all deaths from all causes.

The low risk group is only 17% of the adult population aged 30–59, so our combined target groups include 83% of the people

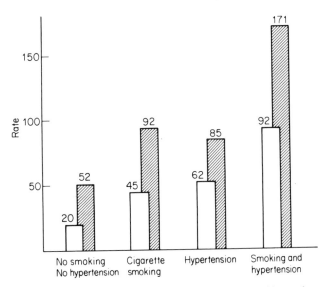

Fig. 7.1 Combined effects of plasma cholesterol, cigarette smoking and hypertension on the risk of coronary heart disease. □ = Plasma cholesterol 'not high'; ▨ = plasma cholesterol 'high'. Ten-year rates per 1000 for first major coronary heart disease events in men aged 30 to 59 years at entry (Stamler & Epstein 1972). (Reproduced with permission from: *The Journal of the Royal Society of Physicians*).

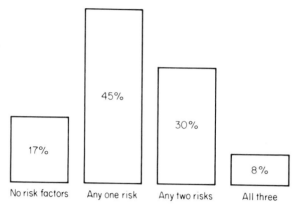

Fig. 7.2 Presence of three risk factors in 7342 US white males aged 30–59. The three risk factors were: blood total cholesterol >6.5 mmol (250 mg)/dl; diastolic pressure >90 mmHg; and any current cigarette smoking.

in this age band in the average practice. If we were to concentrate our efforts only on the 8% with all three risks, we would be ignoring four-fifths of all the coronary events that will occur in the other risk groups. There seems to be no real alternative to tackling the entire middle-aged population, starting at age 30.

However, the results of such a generous definition could be good. For people with more than one major risk factor, subtraction of any one of them seems to have a disproportionately great effect in reducing risk. This is particularly important where smoking is involved, because for coronary disease at least, it is easier to remove completely than is high blood cholesterol, and it now seems very doubtful whether reduction of high blood pressure has much effect.

MORE AND MORE FOR FEWER AND FEWER?

Coping with the consequences of such a Pandora's box presents opportunities to the medical entrepreneur in a private market, whose work is limited only by the willingness and ability of customers to pay; if the job suddenly becomes vastly more complex and time-consuming than was at first thought, this only means that a more comprehensive service will be offered to fewer people, leaving more of the market to competitors. For a market system, people who cannot or will not pay are an inconvenient after-thought, and are then more or less (but always less) provided for by supplementing the market with some spartan state charity, meanly and incompletely delivered.

For GPs working in the NHS, aiming to deliver effective care to the whole population as a human right, development of this more complex model has terrifying consequences for workload. In a society committed to retreat it is hardly surprising that acceptance is slow, implementation slower still, and serious Government support almost undetectably small. In these circumstances there is understandable reluctance to transcend the more modest demands of a high risk strategy.

REAL AND SUPPOSED ADVANTAGES OF A HIGH RISK STRATEGY

The arguments usually deployed in favour of high risk strategies really boil down to this; everyone, care-givers, Government, and patients alike, can continue much as usual, speeding up a bit if they care to, but without important changes in structure, resources, or concepts of disease.

However, as a point of departure rather than arrival, a modified high risk strategy could have one huge real advantage over mass strategies as hitherto conceived. This is that concentration on high risk groups is a natural and relatively easy next step for doctors, nurses, and the populations they serve, all of whom are accustomed to think in terms of care for a sick minority rather than health conservation for everyone. It allows us to start from where we are, with the people we have.

The mass strategies so far on offer have, with few exceptions, ignored the existence of doctors and nurses already in the field, most of whom could probably be mobilised to implement them if they were helped by better organisation, staffing, and a little additional training. Preventive and so-called curative medicine are not opposed alternatives; the best of both could be unified in the concept of anticipatory care.

ANTICIPATORY CARE

Anticipatory care simply means organising to seek out the most likely causes of future breakdown, and the most effective actions to avoid them, at every patient contact. It accepts the consulting patterns we have now as a social reality whose form can be changed only slowly, but which could acquire a more effective content through informed medical and nursing initiative. The material foundation of this policy is the fact that risk factor control before organ damage generally requires cheap, simple, delegable, labour-intensive techniques applied to very large numbers of people (though in a personalised way), rather than the costly, complex, specialised and technologised care of a smaller number after organ damage has already occurred; stitches in time save nine.

Stated this way the argument seems self-evident and unlikely to arouse much opposition; indeed, as long as it remains only an argument rather than a guide to new investment, it has universal support, above all from the Government. In fact however, any attempt to put it into effect runs into fierce resistance: from Governments, when they realise that it implies health care for everyone, not only those getting it now (for example, for the roughly 50% of all diabetics and hypertensives not receiving any regular medical attention), and that ineffective and perfunctory care for the many, together with dazzling technological triumphs for a few, is both popular with the press and cheap for the taxpayer; from specialists, who fear either that their departments will be swamped with unmanageable numbers or that new investment will go to primary care rather than hospitals; and from GPs in search of a quiet life.

MUST ORGANISED PREVENTION LEAD TO BUREAUCRACY?

The entirely reasonable fears of GPs that anticipatory care will lead to a monotonously pastoral rather than excitingly predatory style of practice in the future, was well expressed by Keith Thompson in 1982:

> much of the attraction of general practice is its unpredictability. Yet more and more doctors can say that at 11.30 on Tuesday they will be doing antenatals, and 3.30 on Wednesday they will be doing a hypertension clinic, and of course they will be doing a good job, carefully making measurements and recording them, maintaining flow charts, issuing prescriptions and adjusting drug doses.
> These doctors are doing preventive medicine, and nothing is more important — and nothing is more dull . . . among the many boring aspects of modern general practice, nothing has spread the mantle of dullness more than screening for hypertension and following it up. . . The trouble with good organisation and the establishment of the clinic for a specific condition is that within the imposed structure, there are fewer possibilities. And the detection of variation at an early stage sets in motion processes which prevent a doctor from ever encountering the 'neglected' case which illustrated the text books in our younger days.

The point is well made and well taken. We have plenty of experience of institutionalised screening and administrative medicine, withered at the root and persisting (apparently forever) because doctors can earn a lot for doing little more than apply their signature. Bureaucracy can infect doctors like anyone else, and is bound to thrive where unexpected events are excluded, in specialised follow-up clinics of the well and almost well. The argument applies just as much to nurses, who are even more likely to be delegated repetitive work without explanation of where it comes from, where it goes to, or how it will be used.

But we are growing up now, and learning to do without the fire-engine medicine which still takes up most undergraduate teaching. Who says human biology, and even more its application in the field, is dull, easy and predictable? Our biggest problem is that it is so complex and difficult, yet must somehow be made simple enough to permit mass application. Bureaucratisation of preventive and anticipatory care is a real danger, but we can prevent it if we really want to by insisting on three principles: continuity of personal care, so that the team sees the consequences of its work in a community it knows; continuity of clinical medicine and nursing, so that no task is allowed to become so specialised that variety and unpredictable patient demand are eliminated; and evaluation by audit of outcomes, which must include measures of both patient-satisfaction and care-provider satisfaction. Optimal care is impossible where efficiency is either absent or maximal.

WILL IT WORK?

The best evidence on this comes from the WHO European multicentre controlled trial of multifactorial prevention of coronary heart disease, whose 6-year findings were published in 1986. The study used 60 881 men aged 40–59 at entry, working in matched pairs of factories, half of which received preventive advice on cholesterol-lowering diet, exercise, and on control of smoking, obesity and blood pressure and the other half provided controls. The participating countries were Belgium, Italy, Poland, and Britain. Pooling the results from all these centres, intervention was associated with a reduction of 6.9% in fatal coronary events, 14.8% in non-fatal events, and 5.3% in deaths from all causes, and the authors concluded that 'advice on risk factor reduction in middle-aged men is effective to the extent that it is accepted and it appears to be safe.'

Despite these encouraging overall results, the large British component had so little success in achieving sustained risk factor control that there was no positive impact at all on coronary events. Overall risk actually rose by 4% in the British workers, compared with a 26% reduction in risk for Italian workers, and changes in morbidity and mortality followed the same pattern. Some of this difference must be attributable to the staffing levels used for health education in the two countries. In Britain one whole-time equivalent (WTE) doctor and one WTE nurse were responsible for 9734 workers, compared with two WTE doctors and one WTE nurse for 3131 workers in Italy, a $4\frac{1}{2}$-fold difference (WHO 1982). This is yet another illustration of the Second Law of Prevention; real outputs are proportional to real inputs. Unfortunately recent British governments seem to be familiar only with the First Law; talking about prevention is cheaper than medical salvage.

The other participating countries worked for and achieved better control, and consequently had better results. Dietary advice stood out as probably the most effective single measure, and blood pressure control was least effective.

STARTING FROM WHERE WE ARE, WITH THE PEOPLE WE HAVE

British GPs and primary care teams which have been attracted to organised care of hypertension are generally aware of the preventive nature of this work, and that it will eventually lead to more comprehensive approaches to prevention. Blood pressure is not the only place to make a start, but at least it has the merit of popularity; it is where most of the most progressive teams are at. They will rightly prefer to do the good job that can be done within the resources now available, than try to build Jerusalem with two bricks and a teaspoonful of cement.

Personalised control of all the main risk factors for premature death, uniting the tasks of public health with those of personal care, is now a possible and necessary aim for all GPs and others who work with them, but it is a line of march rather than an immediate objective. We are considering an entirely new agenda, the details of which will be filled in by several generations of primary health workers; we must accept some point at which to begin, and not expect to arrive in less than a lifetime.

Eventually some court is going to decide that knowledge of a registered patient's blood pressure is a minimum obligation for that person's own doctor, and that GPs who fail to organise to provide this are negligent. That will translate into law what most of us already accept in practice; that were we to find one of our patients stretched out dead from a brain haemorrhage, with no blood pressure ever recorded, we would feel deeply ashamed. We must find all the hidden severe hypertensives on our own stretch of the front.

If we do that job, and go on doing it, we are going to find two or three times as many people with blood pressures high enough to constitute a high relative risk, but not high enough to justify antihypertensive medication. These people can be our starting point for the more effective primary care of the future, when we shall have a National Health Service not just a National Disease Service.

SIX CLASSICAL RISK FACTORS FOR ARTERIAL DISEASE

Many prospective studies of populations have firmly established six classical risk factors; blood pressure, age, sex, family history, cigarette smoking, and serum cholesterol. Measurement of these factors permits definition of subgroups with relatively high risk or coronary heart disease or stroke. Other less potent, more doubtful, or promising but as yet little-understood risk factors have also been defined and will be discussed later in this chapter, but the guts of any serious strategy lie in these six, and the interactions between them.

The most important source of evidence has been the continuing follow-up, now reaching 30 years, of a cohort of over 5000 men and women aged 45–74 at entry, randomly sampled in 1949 from the population of Framingham, Massachusetts. All the main conclusions of this study have been confirmed by other large long-term surveys in the USA, Australia, Britain, and Sweden, as well as by many smaller studies in most parts of the developed world. This evidence is of lasting importance because intervention with antihypertensive drugs is now common enough to interfere with the natural history of hypertension on a population scale, and such studies can no longer be done in industrialised countries. This was not true even in the USA in 1974 when the data presented here were collected, and the explanation by Dr W. B. Kannel (1975a) of why this was so is still interesting:

In the early stages of the Framingham study, our claim that we were studying the natural history was held to be untrue because we reported our findings to the physician responsible for the patient and also notified the patient of any abnormalities we had observed. We found that nothing happens when you do that. Hypertensives remain hypertensive, the obese remain obese, smokers continue to smoke, cholesterol values are just as they were before. It is a complete waste of time to screen and refer patients to practising physicians for intervention, without giving some back-up assistance and some sort of organisation to help the physician cope.

Since then, the era of mass antihypertensive medication has begun almost everywhere, mostly by ad hoc case-finding.

ARTERIAL PRESSURE AS AN INDEPENDENT RISK FACTOR

Figure 7.3 from the Framingham study 18-year follow-up shows relative risks for coronary heart disease, claudication, brain infarction and heart failure for normotensive, borderline, and hypertensive subjects, using systolic blood pressure <140, 140–159, and >160 mmHg as thresholds. At first sight the differences are striking: male coronary heart disease is 250% commoner in hypertensives than normotensives (300% in women), claudication is 86% commoner (350% in women), stroke is 800% commoner (750% times in women), and heart failure is 650% commoner (450% in women).

But if you look at absolute rather than relative risks, the picture is very different. What are the chances of one of these hypertensives (aged 45–74) actually getting one of these complications during 5 years of follow-up? For coronary disease, 12% for men and 6% for women; for claudication, 3% for men and 1% for women; for brain infarction, 2% for both men and women; and for heart failure, 4% for men and 2% for women. Clearly at this very low threshold these risks are not sufficient to justify the lifelong use of antihypertensive drugs, if these drugs themselves introduce risks of the same magnitude, and there is good evidence that they do. Looked at in this way, it is surprising that anyone ever thought medication from this threshold (160/95 mmHg) would lead to a significant net saving of life.

The trouble with this strategy is that it concentrates treatment on single risk factors, within such small population groups that, even if it were fully operated, it could have little effect on the overall burden of cardiovascular disease. Using Framingham data, only 36% of all deaths causally related to systolic pressure

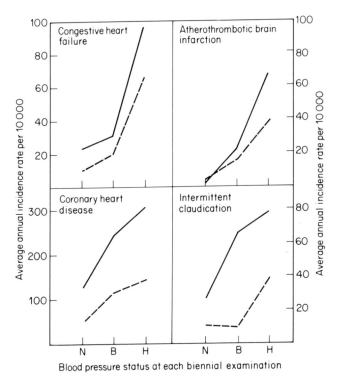

Fig. 7.3 Average annual incidence of cardiovascular disease according to blood pressure status at each biennial examination of men (continuous lines) and women (dashed lines) aged 55–64 at entry into the Framingham study: 18-year follow-up. N = normal; B = borderline; H = hypertensive. (Kannel 1975). (Reproduced with the kind permission of Dr Kannel.)

>140 mmHg occur in the subgroup >180 mmHg; and even of these, two-thirds are coronary deaths which are not preventable by reduction of blood pressure alone. In fact, in middle age there is no systolic or diastolic threshold below which the level of pressure is unrelated to risk. Even in the diastolic range 80–89 mmHg, risk of cardiovascular death is 39% higher than for people with diastolic pressures <80 mmHg (Kannel 1975b).

ARTERIAL PRESSURE AS A COMBINED RISK FACTOR

Now study Figure 7.4, showing the risk of a cardiovascular or cerebrovascular event over 8 years' follow-up for 40-year-old men with a systolic pressure of 165 mmHg, according to the presence of other risk factors. The difference in risk between the bottom and

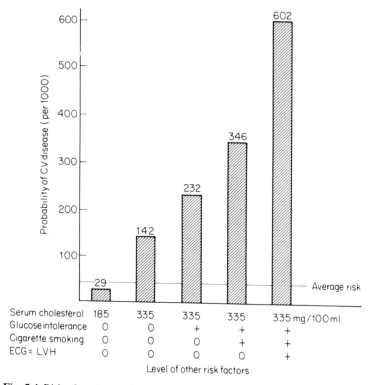

Fig. 7.4 Risk of cardiovascular (CV) disease in an 8-year period at systolic blood pressure of 165 mmHg according to level of other risk factors in 40-year-old men. ECG–LVH = electrocardiogram — left ventricular hypertrophy. Framingham study: 18-year follow-up. (Reproduced with permission, from: *Hypertension, its nature, and treatment (malta Symposium, 1974)*, (CIBA Laboratories, 1975).

top centiles of serum total cholesterol distributions is more than fourfold; glucose intolerance raises it more than sevenfold; cigarette smoking raises it again more than 11-fold, and when there is also ECG evidence of left ventricular hypertrophy, the risk is raised more than 20 times.

Obviously it is absurd to ignore these other risks and concentrate only on treating hypertension, but this is in fact what most of us do; we give priority to blood pressure control and leave the other risks till later, which often means never.

Part of this problem has been how to handle the essentially mathematical conception of multivariate risk. An important development here is the availability of pocket calculators containing a dedicated computer. These give a percentage risk of heart or brain infarction over the next 6 years, based on eight sets of data (sex, age, smoking, diabetes, heart size, systolic pressure, total cholesterol and HDL cholesterol). The underlying algorithm is derived from Framingham data. This is particularly helpful in giving patients feedback on their achievement in reduction of risk when they reduce cholesterol or stop smoking. These calculators cost about $17 in the USA, and are available free in the UK from Pfizer Ltd. to any GP who runs a separate hypertension clinic.

Because the control of other risk factors mainly requires change in behaviour rather than pill-taking, the risks tend never to be tackled at all. Ironically, for coronary prevention (but not for prevention of stroke or heart failure) control of blood pressure has little or no effect, whereas stopping smoking and lowering blood cholesterol by reducing animal fat and increasing fish and vegetable foods can both be very effective. These topics are dealt with more fully in Chapter 14.

Worse still, many of the drugs used to reduce blood pressure tend to raise blood cholesterol and some impair glucose tolerance and promote arrhythmias. This topic is considered fully in Chapters 16 and 17.

CONCLUSIONS

When high blood pressure is already causing symptoms or measurable organ damage, its control should obviously have priority and plans for this may safely ignore other cardiovascular risks, but this applies only to brief initial episodes. In all other situations, and for nearly all work in primary care, hypertension is only one of several possible risk factors, all of which must be taken into account in formulating and negotiating with the patient an intelligent plan for anticipatory care. Blood pressure control is nearly always less important than stopping smoking (because not smoking reduces risk over such a wide range of disease) and control of alcohol problems, and usually less important than reduction of total blood cholesterol by diet and exercise. Obese patients with a history of diabetes in first-degree relatives will also usually reduce cardiovascular risk more by reducing weight than by taking antihypertensive drugs. These points need to be constantly borne in mind. For historical reasons, this book is presented as a discourse on high blood pressure and its treatment, but its hidden agenda is the prevention of arterial disease by control of risk factors, of which hypertension is only one — on present evidence one of the less reversible in most of its effects — and therefore less important.

REFERENCES

Kannel W B 1975a Assessment of hypertension as a predictor of cardiovascular disease in the Framingham study. In: Burley D M, Birdwood G F B, Fryer J H, Taylor S H (eds) Hypertension; its nature and treatment. International Symposium Malta 1974; Ciba Laboratories, Horsham, p 69

Kannel W B 1975b Role of blood pressure in cardiovascular disease: the Framingham study. Angiology 26:1

Stamler J, Epstein F H 1982 Coronary heart disease: risk factors as guides to preventive action. Preventive Medicine 1:27

Thompson K 1982 Are you bored with general practice? General Practitioner (London)

World Health Organization European Collaborative Group 1982 Multifactorial trial in the prevention of coronary heart disease: 2. Risk factor changes at two and four years. European Heart Journal 3:184

World Health Organization European Collaborative Group 1986 European collaborative trial of multifactorial prevention of coronary heart disease: final report of the 6-year results. Lancet i:869

8

Case-finding and screening

Because high blood pressure at any level rarely causes symptoms, it must be looked for. Everyone has a blood pressure, and its value is unknown until it has been measured. No British court has yet found a GP guilty of negligence because (I quote a real example, settled out of court for a large sum in favour of the widow) his registered patient, a man of 45, died of an unheralded cerebral haemorrhage with no record of his blood pressure despite over a dozen consultations for various reasons over the previous ten years; but it is only a matter of time. Meanwhile we are surely under a moral if not a legal obligation to record blood pressure at least once in every 5-year span for every registered adult in our practice, if we are to prevent tragedies of this kind.

To achieve this requires organisation, and what would at one time have been called screening; the organised application of a standard diagnostic procedure to as many as possible of a defined group of the population, with or without presenting complaints.

WHY NOT SCREENING?

The idea of screening for clinical rather than research purposes began in the early 1960s, as a result of two developments: new diagnostic and information technology, which made it possible to generate and handle diagnostic data on a large scale; and post-war epidemiology of non-infective disease, which provided a conceptual framework through which strategies for mass diagnosis and intervention could be developed.

Clinical screening then developed in three entirely different directions. In the USA, and to a smaller extent in other fee-paid medical care systems, the idea of earlier diagnosis and earlier treatment by detection of presymptomatic departures from supposed normal values was embraced with enthusiasm, and generous investments of staff and equipment were made. The only British experience of this kind of screening is that offered outside the NHS by the British United Provident Association (BUPA), which both assists and irritates GPs from time to time by sending multiple-risk printouts and biochemical profiles about their NHS patients. Because screening of this kind is based on fees, large proportions of the population at risk without insurance cover are omitted and its effectiveness cannot be evaluated on epidemiological lines. As such schemes are self-financing they have attracted little criticism, except for their possible effect in raising expectations of NHS patients which cannot be met. For the medical entrepreneurs themselves, the idea of simultaneously assisting the public health and filling their own pockets has been both a powerful spur to enterprise, and an effective cure for doubt.

The second type of screening was developed experimentally, usually with academic and Government backing, to evaluate the effectiveness and efficiency of screening before public demand might make it a mandatory and expensive addition to public medical services. An early example was the Varmland project in Sweden. Epidemiologists and community physicians developed the methodology of these schemes, generally with little regard for existing systems of primary care (a notable exception was the programme near Glasgow developed by Hawthorn et al (1974)). Generally, negative conclusions were quickly accepted for non-commercial primary care (Wilson & Jungner 1968; Hart 1975). Two leading epidemiologists concluded that the case for screening for hypertension was not made (Sackett 1974; Sackett & Holland 1975). Reluctantly, they conceded only that GPs might usefully continue case-finding, which as they described it meant only continued standard practice.

Thirdly, a few GPs, mainly in Britain, Scandinavia, and the Netherlands, made constructive use of their autonomous care of defined populations to set up their own screening programmes (Hart 1970; Coope 1974; Pedersen & Nielsen 1975; van der Feen 1975; Lindholm 1984), and large schemes for organised case-finding with planned follow-up were launched in some countries of the Eastern bloc, notably the German Democratic Republic. Screening by these groups differed from traditional case-finding in aiming to reach whole populations, to audit results, and generally to become less dependent on patient-initiative (reactive), and to initiate planned action themselves (proactive). The few schemes in western Europe, begun by enthusiasts, have, so far as I know, all prospered, with steadily improving results in terms of high response, sustained reductions in blood pressure in identified hypertensives, and low drop-out rates. I know of only three which have published these results (Van der Feen 1976; Hart 1978; Lindholm 1984) but these were as good as, or better than, the best results of hospital clinics, and unlike them were tackling a much bigger and more important task, the control of moderate and severe hypertension in entire populations at risk.

DOES CASE-FINDING WORK?

Doubt remained, however, whether these results could be achieved by GPs on a mass scale. A large study by the department of community medicine at St Thomas's hospital compared ascertainment and control of hypertension in co-operating general practices randomly allocated to assisted screening or to customary case-finding, without organisation or audit (D'Souza et al 1976). This showed uniformly poor results in both groups, and has ever since been quoted as evidence that screening in primary care is ineffective.

Certainly it was ineffective in the practices studied, but GPs who continued the struggle (and it was struggle) for effective organised screening and follow-up despite these results have been rewarded by the now mounting evidence of effective work on these lines in a growing minority of practices throughout Britain. Screening for hypertension with audited follow-up was the most commonly preferred theme for members of the RCGP who took part in the College's 'Quality Initiative' in 1984–1985. There is now no question that this is not only the most effective method of controlling moderate and severe hypertension in the general population, but also the only one that is feasible in British conditions, because the scale of the problem is far beyond the resources of hospitals.

What then was wrong with the St Thomas's trial? It evidently lacked the enthusiasm evident in all successful accounts of primary care screening. If enthusiasm is or was absent in many practices, action is required to change them, because evidently enthusiasm is an essential ingredient of effective mass work. Perhaps the fault lay in outside rather than inside leadership; successful teams set their own goals, and their own measures of achievement. Historically, good science and scientific innovation have been passionate activities, with warm hearts as well as cool heads.

AD HOC CASE-FINDING

Both academic epidemiologists and GPs who hope for painless progress cling to the view that if we all practise good clinical medicine it will just happen, without any special organisation. This is the initial attraction of the case-finding idea. About three-quarters of any population consults a GP at least once a year for something, so all we have to do is measure blood pressures in all these people. I well remember trying to interest a local consultant physician in our original Glyncorrwg blood pressure screening campaign in 1968; I was very excited at having achieved virtually 100% coverage, but he put me properly in my place with the remark that he had always measured blood pressure in all his patients, and was surprised that I had not done the same.

However attractive this policy may appear, it seldom works, at any rate by itself. GPs who resolve to record blood pressures of all their patients at every reasonable opportunity have consistently found, when they audit their work, that they are actually doing no better than before; the proportion of patients with no pressure recorded remains exactly the same (Neville & McKellican 1984; Fleming et al 1985). Experienced GPs know well why this is so. Case-finding is no different from most other policy decisions in general practice; no theory is ever transformed into practice until specific responsibilities are allocated, measurable targets are set, and their attainment is verified some time later.

There is nothing intrinsically wrong with case-finding: indeed it is the obvious and I think most effective and economical way to begin, but its apparent simplicity and painlessness are deceptive. It has to be planned, organised, and verified if it is to become anything more than a good idea inside your head. It is easy to think in this way if, like my consultant, you work in a large medical care factory with lots of junior staff and nurses to implement your excellence on your behalf. It is not so easy if, as nearly all GPs do, you work in what more nearly resembles a small cobbler's shop, where nothing seems to get done unless you do it yourself. The change required is not in clinical medicine, but in resources and organisation.

SCREENING THE RECORDS

Having decided to stop relying on doing everything the same but better, your first step will be to screen not the patients, but the records. You will need to know how many people have never had a blood pressure recorded at all, how many treated hypertensives you are already following up (and perhaps how many of them were started on treatment on questionable evidence), how many known hypertensives appear to have lapsed from supervision and perhaps from medication, and how many people have had no blood pressure recorded during the past 5 years.

All that is a stern test of the quality of your records. Almost certainly you will find much fewer data than you expected. Perhaps you or your partners have recorded only what you considered abnormal findings, and perhaps it will be very difficult to understand from the records whether the patient is still on medication, and if so, what. How much information is there about other risk factors, such as smoking, blood cholesterol and obesity? Are weights recorded? Probably many are, but are heights recorded? Probably almost none; when you are reviewing individual patients rather than their records, you can tell if they're fat just by looking at them, but for record review without visible patients, you must have the heights.

You will want to decide which age and sex groups you are going to go for, or go for first. Practices which have not screened in an organised way invariably have a lot more hypertensive women recognised and on treatment than men (Keith Hodgkin continues to report a male: female ratio of 1:5 in the fifth edition of his book (1985)), although hypertension has a higher prevalence in men than women until late middle age, and treatment of men is more effective in preventing organ damage, at least in mild hypertension (MRC 1985).

The best way to go about this is to draw a small random sample of records in the age or sex group you have chosen, and do a really thorough analysis of these before making any further plans. You will then know what you are up against. Studies of randomly sampled practice records, even from practices already well ahead in anticipatory care, generally show very incomplete data and an enormous amount of work still to be done; one audit of five practices in the Oxford region (Mant & Phillips 1986) showed the range of completeness of risk-data recording seen in Table 8.1. From data like these you can calculate roughly how much time it will take to cover the whole population at risk in your selected age range, with your present staff resources. You may want to make decisions about increasing your staff, or about changing your record system. The 'you' referred to in this chapter might be a good practice manager.

Table 8.1 Percentage of 2000 randomly sampled patient records (age 25–64 years) from five practices, including data on cardiovascular risk factors

Risk factor	Mean	Range
Blood pressure	65%	54–73%
Smoking	50%	19–77%
Alcohol	12%	8–16%
Height	20%	2–45%
Weight	33%	17–53%
Diet	7%	1–14%
Exercise	3%	0–9%
Occupation	42%	21–68%

TAGGING THE RECORDS

Having identified the records with missing information, you will need a tagging system to make the omissions obvious next time these particular subjects visit your centre, so that the person responsible for measuring blood pressure or collecting other data can know when to do so.

With Lloyd-George records the simplest way to do this is to get a local do-it-yourself shop to cut up a coloured resin-laminate sheet into a number of slats, long enough to stick up out of the record envelopes but short enough not to scrape the top of their shelves or drawers, and numerous enough to have one in every record that needs it. As blood pressures are measured, the slats are taken out so that the work is not duplicated. When one job is finished you can use the slats for the next. This is the method we used in Glyn-corrwg in 1968; we converted to A4 folders in 1977.

With A4 folders it is more difficult; in fact this is the only convincing argument I have heard in defence of a record system which was devised for the general practice in 1915, and is still in use in 1986. There is no way to attach any removable signal to any part of an A4 folder which will not come off in the rough and tumble of office consultation or home visits. The simplest and therefore best method is probably to make one diagonal stroke on the outside of each record with a felt pen for those who need data collecting, and to cross this out with an opposing stroke when the job has been done. An alternative, which has apparently worked in some practices, is to write (or rubber-stamp) an instruction to the next doctor who sees the patient, thus:

> BP, SMOKING, WEIGHT AND HEIGHT
> NEXT TIME PLEASE

The capacity of both my colleagues and myself to ignore or find excuses for evading such a request has taught me that in my practice at least, this doesn't work, perhaps because it is seen only by someone opening the record at the start of a consultation, which nearly always means a doctor. On the whole, nurses and office staff have a more organised approach to their work than doctors, and are less likely to ignore a protocol once it has been agreed and understood.

BOXED CARD INDEXES

As possible hypertensives are identified, and actual hypertensives are verified by repeated readings, cases found must be listed so that active follow-up and audit are possible. The traditional alternative, simply to tell patients they have high blood pressure and leave it to them to return without any means of recognising default, will soon lead to re-establishment of the situation as it was before you began trying to rationalise it. This is particularly true early on in the management of newly discovered cases, because several sessions are usually needed before patients fully understand that they are not ill, but do need lifelong follow-up, and usually lifelong medication.

The answer is simple: set up a boxed card index, organised into the months of the year so that as patients are seen they move into the next 3 month slot (or whatever interval you have chosen). Having once set up the box, it is particularly important to ensure that subsequent new cases (after the initial excitement of the screening campaign) get into the pipeline. Patients should also be asked to contact the receptionist themselves if they ever find they have been out of contact for more than 3 months; this is a useful fail-safe device against inevitable organisational failures.

CONTACTING THE POPULATION

Traditionally, the only way GPs have tried to reach their patients as a group has been to put up a notice in the waiting room. As we all know, such notices can be virtually guaranteed to produce no response whatever.

If you are planning to contact the whole of your population aged between 35 and 64, you will be having quite an impact on your local community, and you should think about the public relations aspect of your work in a positive way. In urban practice, where several possibly competing practices interpenetrate the population, it may be useful to contact some of these colleagues and see if they are interested in doing more or less the same thing at the same time. If they are, it will be easier to have a fairly high public profile, with posters in shops and write-ups in local papers to advertise meetings for your patients where they can come with their families to hear about your plans and ask questions. Times are changing with regard to medical advertising, and serious complaints on that score are unlikely.

In Glyncorrwg we are fortunate in having a real community, where people know and care about one another. Public meetings on health questions are held two or three times a year, and are usually well attended, with audiences of 30–60. Where consultants have been prepared to come out and meet their patients and discuss the work of their hospital departments this has been much appreciated, but GPs generally have more experience of communication with local people, and have the huge advantage of anecdotal experiences shared with their audience. Explanations of cardiovascular risk factors given to local public meetings are an important and neglected way of supplementing individual patient education, and have a lasting effect by recruiting local opinion-formers to your cause and giving them more reliable information than they are likely to have picked up by themselves.

WHAT ABOUT NON-RESPONDENTS?

A question always brought up at both public and professional meetings is the degree to which we are justified in pushing diagnosis and care on people who have not asked for it and may not want it. This often used to be raised as a largely imaginary obstacle by people anxious to find enough difficulties to justify their own inaction, but that is now uncommon; the question is important and should be taken seriously. For reasons I cannot understand, it seems to worry GPs in Denmark and the Netherlands much more than in the UK.

Another fear commonly expressed is that screening increases the labelling of apparently well people as having a disease, creating feelings of insecurity and perhaps increasing work absence. Work with Canadian steelworkers by Haynes et al (1978) supported this view. Van Weel in the Netherlands (1985) found no evidence that labelling as a hypertensive had any effect on subsequent consulting behaviour other than the direct effects of hypertension management. My own view is that, providing that both care-givers and care-receivers fully understand that neither hypertension nor any other cardiovascular risk factor is a disease in its own right, and provided that doctors have no economic incentive to create dependence, any such effect is more than discounted by the greater confidence engendered by any properly organised health maintenance system. This view is supported by the results of the MRC study on the psychological effects of the mild hypertension trial (1977).

There is no doubt that a majority of people would like a more outgoing and more preventively oriented service, but the minority who do not like, or do not think they would like, this style of care, should be recognised and allowed for in all plans for screening. Anne Cartwright's study (1967) of experience of general practice in a large random sample of the general population in many parts of England in 1964 found that nearly two-thirds of patients interviewed would like some kind of regular check-up on their health, with a higher proportion of younger than older patients, so that one would expect this to be a growing trend. The main reason for not wanting check-ups was not from worries about lost independence, but because many people did not believe such check-ups were effective, and in 1964 there was perhaps something to be said for that view. A minority was actively hostile to proactive screening: 5% because they feared discovery of serious illness and preferred not to know, 7% because they actively disliked going to doctors, and 4% for poorly formulated reasons.

It is disappointing that in her follow-up study on the same lines in 1977 (Cartwright & Anderson 1981), Cartwright hardly touched on this question, though it is now much more a live issue and there is far more interest in it among GPs. Since the publication of the RCGP reports on prevention, particularly the one on prevention of arterial disease (1981), there has been accelerating interest in preventive work, and more general recognition that an anticipatory population approach can and should be flexible enough to allow for a wide variety of personal attitudes.

Experience in Glyncorrwg suggests that when a systematic anticipatory style of care has been developed over a decade or more, it is almost universally accepted. We have about 10 (out of 1700) patients clearly identified as people who reject medical care of any kind unless they are seriouly ill, though all but one of these has been willing to see a nurse at home about once every 5 years for a blood pressure check.

WORLD WITHOUT END

Proactive care, with an organised case-finding approach, cannot be limited to a search for only one risk, and inevitably leads to a much wider definition of the GP's role. As this role is obviously narrowing in some other important directions, for example childbirth and all conditions requiring specialised skills, I see no reason to fear the lurid scenario painted by Ivan Illich and other dystopian prophets, who claim to fear that doctors will medicalise the whole world. As long as we can avoid a historical retreat to fee-paid care, the limiting factor for medical imperialism will be the time and effort required to extend and maintain our frontier. No one who has actually undertaken a serious screening programme in general practice will be anything but sceptical about new suggestions for apparently simple things which should be done for everybody. Unquestionably, this approach will grow, but in our care system I doubt if it will do so any faster than the evidence allows.

REFERENCES

Cartwright A 1967 Patients and their doctors; a study of general practice. Routledge and Kegan Paul, London

Cartwright A, Anderson R 1981 General practice revisited; a second study of patients and their doctors. Tavistock Publications, London

Coope J 1974 A screening clinic for hypertension in general practice. Journal of the Royal College of General Practitioners 24:161

D'Souza M F, Swan A V, Shannon D J 1976 A long-term controlled trial of screening for hypertension in general practice. Lancet i:1228

Editorial 1985 Quality in general practice. Policy statement 2. Royal College of General Practitioners, London

Fleming D M, Lawrence M S T, Cross K W 1985 List size, screening methods, and other characteristics of practices in relation to preventive care. British Medical Journal 291:869

Hart J T 1970 Semicontinuous screening of a whole community for hypertension. Lancet ii:223

Hart J T 1975 Screening in primary care. In: Hart C R (ed) Screening in general practice. Churchill-Livingstone, Ediburgh, p 17

Hart J T 1980 Future strategies of hypertension control by age. In Coope J (ed) Hypertension in primary care: an international symposium held at Reykjavik, Iceland, April 1978. RCGP, London: pp 11–12

Hawthorn V M, Greaves D A, Beavers D G 1974 Blood pressure in a Scottish town. British Medical Journal iii:600

Haynes R B, Sackett D L, Taylor D W et al 1978. Increased absenteeism from work after detection and labelling of hypertensive patients. New England Journal of Medicine 299:741

Hodgkin K 1984 Towards earlier diagnosis; a guide to primary care. Churchill Livingstone, Edinburgh

Lindholm L 1984 Hypertension and its risks: epidemiological studies in Swedish primary health care. Department of Community Health Sciences, Dalby

Mant D, Phillips A 1986 Can the prevalence of disease risk factors be assessed from general practice records? British Medical Journal 292:102

Medical Research Council Working Party on Mild-to-moderate Hypertension 1977 Randomised controlled trial of treatment for mild hypertension: design and pilot trial. British Medical Journal i:1437

Medical Research Council Working Party 1985 MRC trial of treatment of mild hypertension: principal results. British Medical Journal 291:97

Neville R G, McKellican J F 1984 Audit on hypertension management in general practice. Family Practice 1:168

Pedersen O L, Nielsen E G 1975 Screening for hypertension in general practice. Danish Medical Bulletin 22:18

RCGP Working Party on Prevention of Arterial Disease 1981 Prevention of arterial disease in general practice. Reports from general practice 19. Royal College of General Practitioners, London

Sackett D L 1974 Screening for disease; cardiovascular diseases. Lancet ii:1189

Sackett D L, Holland W W 1975 Controversy in detection of disease. Lancet ii:357

Van der Feen J A E 1975 Hypertension and the general practitioner: a challenge. Huisarts en Wetenschap 18:406

Van der Feen J A E 1976 A follow-up study on a general study (screening) of hypertension in general practice. Huisarts en Wetenschap 19:266

Van Weel C 1985 Does labelling and treatment for hypertension increase illness behaviour? Family Practice 2:147

Wilson J M G, Jungner G 1968 Principles and practice of screening for disease. Public Health Papers no 34. WHO, Geneva

9

Record systems

As you collect your new data, you will want to put them somewhere that is readily accessible for future management, and which involves the least possible amount of duplication. This is difficult with A4 paper, and almost impossible with Lloyd-George records.

STRUCTURING LLOYD-GEORGE RECORDS

If you are sticking to Lloyd-George, a special card is essential. Several reasonably good designs are available free from the various antihypertensive drug firms, but none of them ever seem to be quite right for what you personally want for your particular team. As you can get unlimited supplies of NHS continuation cards free, you can easily design your own pattern, and submit it to pilot trial. Then, and only then (you will certainly want to revise it in the light of pilot experience), you can take it to a local printer and get a few thousand done at small cost. If you decide to have a patient-held card (discussed below), this can carry a few sentences of educational material, reminding the patient yet again that hypertension is not a disease and rarely causes symptoms.

If your special cards are not patient-held, they are going to take up more space in the Lloyd-George envelope. You may decide to take this opportunity to replace your existing two-dimensional envelopes with gusseted envelopes, to accommodate the larger records which will inevitably begin to accumulate.

CONVERSION TO A4 RECORDS

The work of converting to A4 is appalling. It takes about 3 minutes simply to do Stage 1, assembling the folder and entering identification data; that alone comes to 100 hours of work for a list of 2000. There are few things worse than a practice stuck in half-conversion, so once started, Stage 1 must be completed as quickly as possible.

Stage 2 is to get out the hospital correspondence, laboratory reports, and so on, iron them flat, cull out the rubbish, get them into date order, punch a pair of holes in them, and then put them on to the folding prongs on the right-hand side of the folder. Depending on the amount of hospital referral and direct-access investigation, this will take another 3–5 minutes for each folder, and another 150 hours or so, but again the work can be delegated to office staff.

Stage 3 is the real problem, and in my opinion it cannot be delegated; making problem summaries, and sorting out a repeat prescribing list. Hannay and Mitchell (1985) in the Glasgow university teaching practice found it took 25 minutes for the average patient, working out at 833 hours for an average list of 2000. I am surprised that it took as long as this and would have guessed a lower figure, but when I did Stage 3 I didn't keep track of the time taken. Certainly it took up most evenings for about a year, but the quality of care thereafter was transformed; all our patients now have full updated lists of major clinical problems, and we wonder now how we ever managed without them (the answer is, of course, that we tolerated a much lower standard of practice). This task too can be put off, though not for ever, by shoving Lloyd-George unread into the left-hand side pocket, to wait until you have time to go through both it and the correspondence, to extract a comprehensible story which must at some time be verified with the patient. For blood pressure and coronary risk screening it is possible to ignore this, and push on to Stage 2, if you decide to combine conversion to A4 with the beginning of screening; the work will be harder, but there will be far less duplication than if you put off A4 conversion to a later and separate time.

One still occasionally hears it said that conversion to A4 is a waste of time because the task will be bypassed by computerised records. On the contrary, those who have not converted to a structured record will find a computer almost impossible to use. If you can restructure within the constraints of the traditional Lloyd-George record, good luck to you. I doubt if this is possible anywhere with a heavy burden of serious organic disease, where many records already look as ill as the patients they represent.

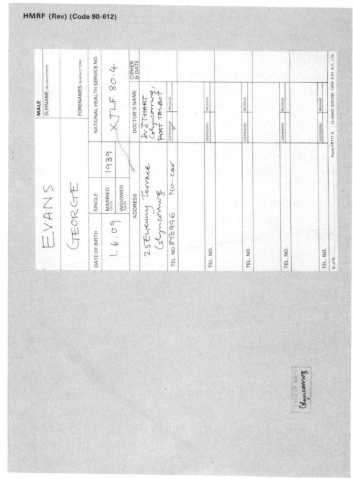

Fig. 9.1 Front outside folder, A4.

STRUCTURING A4 RECORDS

The page and information sequence we use at Glyncorrwg (Fig. 9.1) works well and resembles most of the other A4 systems I have seen:

Front outside folder
Surname, maiden name
Forenames (underline name used)
Address with postcode
Telephone number; indicate if no phone

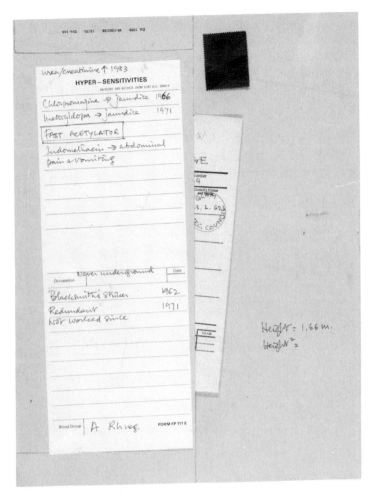

Fig. 9.2 Front inside folder.

Front inside folder
Drug reactions. Use this not only for serious reactions, but any experience you do not want to repeat uselessly, e.g. *'nifedipine → headache'* or *'beta-blockers don't work'*. Also add evidence of renal or hepatic failure, or continuous medication which could complicated prescribing, e.g. anticoagulants or MAO inhibitors.

Current employment, previous employment and skills.

You can see from Figure 9.2 that we also use the inside of the front half of the folder for a square red sticker on which we indicate when (which year) a blood pressure measurement is due. As contraceptive pill-takers are seen every 3 months for a blood pressure check, we write 'pill' on the square at the bottom right corner for these women, and as a convenient extension of this, whatever other method of contraception is in use; intrauterine device, sheath, cap, coitus interruptus, sterilisation, hysterectomy, vasectomy, infertile, hoping for the best, or trying for baby. We think we ought to be interested in where every sexually active

National Health Service Number

Surname (Block Letters): EVANS

Forenames (Block Letters): GEORGE

SUMMARY OF IMPORTANT ILLNESSES AND INVESTIGATIONS

Address: 25 EWENNY TCE

Date of Birth: 1.6.09

Date	
	Smoker 0 (was 15)
	Father d. 49 stroke
	Mother d. 73 heart
1954	impotence
1964	3 jejunal diverticulae ? insignificant
1967	Transient (R) hemiparesis → recognition mean BP $\frac{210}{127}$
	Rx ever since
1971	Obstructive jaundice, probably ∵ methyldopa
	Duodenal ulcer shown Ba meal
	laparotomy showed ulcer eroding pancreas
	Polya gastrectomy
	Sudden hearing loss (L) ear ? cause
1974	Polycythaemia
	Heart failure with atrial fibrillation
1981	Obesity BMI 29 → mild diabetes. Fasting BS 8.6.
1983	Impaired renal function urea ↑ 9.3 creatinine ↑ 148
1984	Deafaid
1985	Stomal ulcer → haematemesis & melaena

Form FP111G

Fig. 9.3 Summary sheet.

woman fits in this pattern: another example of the practical impossibility of restricting management to blood pressure alone.

Below this we enter metric height and height squared, for calculation of body mass index.

Blue summary sheet (Fig. 9.3)
Identification data again; unless this information is entered on every sheet and the sheets are numbered, you won't know who they refer to when, sooner or later, they will have come adrift.

Age and cause of death of parents and siblings. Family history of coronary disease, stroke and diabetes.

Smoking status; just 'smokes' or 'smokes 0'.

Parity

Down the left-hand margin, year plus important events. These must be reasonably firm judgements, including such ambiguities as 'recurrent severe back pain? cause'. They should include major social events such as separation and bereavement. Inevitably, every practice will have some special inclusions or omissions of its own with regard to what should go into an events summary. Down the right-hand margin, results of major investigations, whether positive or negative.

Green sheet, designed for pathology and X-ray reports
We use this as a repeat prescribing sheet. If the receptionist or dispenser date-stamps every repeat prescription, this is a help in checking compliance.

White or pink continuation sheets (Fig. 9.4)
We are currently fitting the hypertension clinic encounters to the same pattern as all other encounters, using the Weed SOAP formula (Weed 1969):

S subjective; what the patient says
O objective; what the doctor finds
A assessment; what the doctor thinks
P plan; what the doctor decides to do about it

We find SOAP useful in introducing a recognisable pattern, and it makes it easier for someone else to find his or her way around the record, bearing in mind that planned care means that records are used much more for reviewing information in the patient's

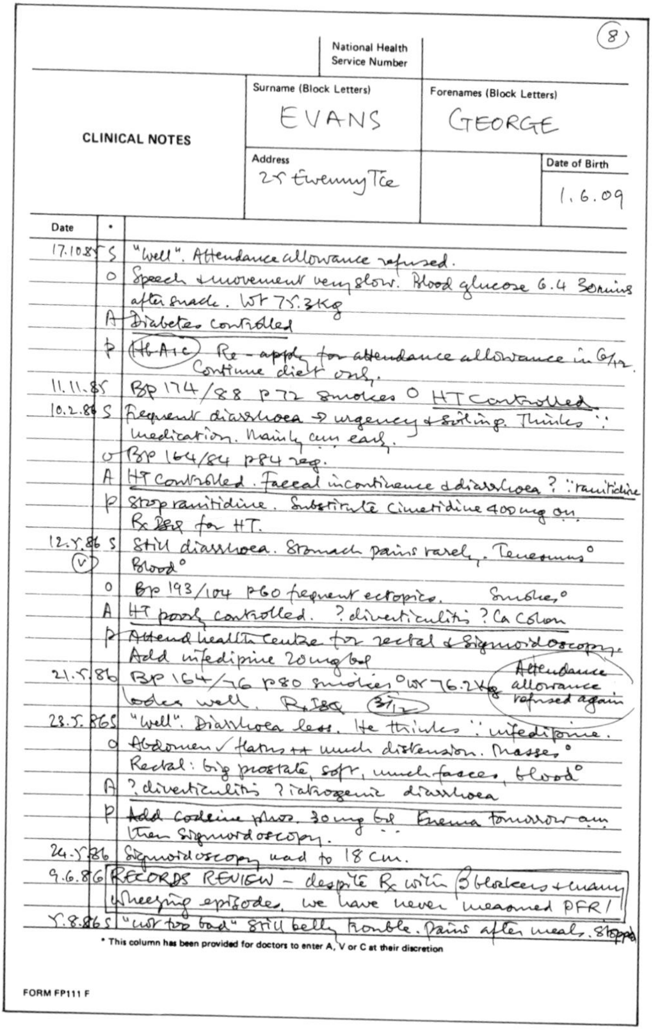

Fig. 9.4 Continuation sheet.

absence. If the patient starts off on a completely different subject, you just start another SOAP; sometimes there are two or three.

Hospital and other correspondence and diagnostic reports
These are filed together, latest news on top.

Yellow immunisation and screening data sheet
This works well for immunisations. As a cumulative data sheet

it is badly designed and we rarely use it, unless a new patient arrives with a lot of previous data. Then it is a useful place to jot down sequences of weights or blood pressures.

Inside back folder:
We don't use this for anything. Data entered on the folder have to be copied whenever the outer folder has begun to fall apart and needs replacement. Because of mean materials and official incapacity to understand that, unlike hospital records, GP records should last a lifetime through wind, snow, rain, and spilt cups of coffee, about 25% of our record folders have had to be replaced after only 8 years. When Britain really was poor, some of the Lloyd-George envelopes were made of a fabric-reinforced high-quality paper which lasted 40 years or more. Perhaps this material needs to be rediscovered.

Outside back folder: ditto.
Unquestionably, A4 makes life richer, but it also makes management more complex, time-consuming, and uncertain. At last it is possible to record intelligently and accessibly at least a little of the extraordinary biological and social complexity, ambiguity and unpredictability of real lives; whereas Lloyd-George restricts us to a more manageable procrustean cot, cramping out everything except a cocksure mnemonic caricature of the patient. This can hardly be corrected, even by hospital reports that contradict it, because as these become bulkier and more difficult to cram into the bag, we become more and more reluctant to take them out and read them.

Over half of all Scottish GPs have converted to A4, compared with about 5% in England and Wales. Why?

NUMERIC FLOW CHARTS

I have never used numeric flow charts and am not convinced of their advantage. They always entail either writing data down twice — bad for staff morale and often fatal to good record keeping because one or the other figure gets missed — or they entail isolating all hypertension-related data from the general record, so that consultations about other problems may be carried on in ignorance of what is going on at the blood pressure clinic. True, the doctor has only to lift the page to find out what is going on in the other department of the file, but in my experience this will seldom be done in practice. Perhaps a more serious criticism is that rows or columns of figures are difficult to follow intelligently; decisions still tend to be based only on the evidence of the most recent entry.

GRAPHIC FLOW CHARTS

Though there is little in favour of numeric flow charts, graphic charts are a different matter. Indeed, I suspect this is the only way to get doctors to pay as much attention to systolic as they do to diastolic pressures — a long-standing and serious problem. They also have the immense advantage that patients can see and understand what is going on, and often can help to relate this to the pattern of medication, and particularly to compliance with medication.

So why do we so seldom do them? All the Glyncorrwg patients have a simple fine-graded graph sheet in their record, but these are only updated about once in 2 years, and therefore serve no useful purpose in management; the work is done for research and teaching rather than patient management, though I have no doubt of the advantage of using this method routinely. The answer probably is that it is one more little thing to do which is not absolutely necessary, we are always short of time, and we have never seriously incorporated it in our protocol. When our blood pressure records are fully computerised, the problem will vanish.

PATIENT-HELD CO-OPERATION CARDS

This again is something I have never done but theoretically approve of, and like graphic flow charts, I suspect its time will come when we have full computerisation. Again, the difficulty lies in duplication; if patients hold the one and only record, then the 10–15% that will be lost (judging from experience of antenatal co-operation cards) will be really serious. If they hold duplicate cards, all data will have to be entered at least twice. Otherwise the idea has everything to be said for it, and would probably improve patient understanding and therefore compliance.

RUBBER STAMPS

This cheap and simple device (Fig. 9.5) can serve two useful functions. Firstly, it prints out the set of data you have decided on for standard operations at screening, detection, and follow-up (you

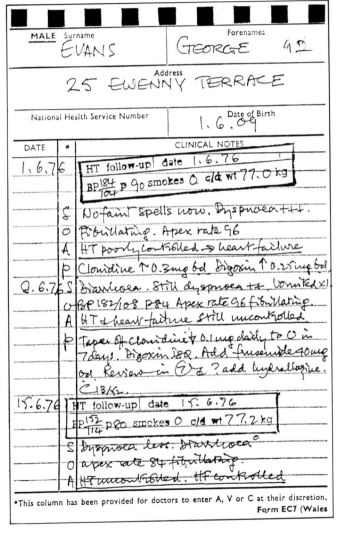

Fig. 9.5 Rubber stamps in use on Lloyd-George system.

need one for each). Secondly, it alerts users of the medical record to the patient's status in relation to the screening programme (screened, detected, or followed-up) in a more effective way than coloured tags on the outside of the record, however prominently these are displayed.

Devices of this sort sound clever but are rarely used for long in general sessions, because their use is too infrequent. When you actually want them they have disappeared under the rest of the desk jumble, unless you are prepared to advertise yourself as a rubber stamp doctor by having an array of them on a stand. They are more useful in an organised screening and follow-up programme, particularly if you set up a mini-clinic. Then you know they will be used, probably by a nurse, and can make sure they are always available in your clinic package.

COMPUTERISED INFORMATION SYSTEMS

The computer scene is more stable now than it was in 1979 when the first edition of this book was written. Hardware prices continue to fall, though more slowly, and as software costs are rising, there is no longer much to be gained in financial terms by waiting. There is little prospect of Government funding in the near future, and the possible demise of item of service payments would make them even more costly to practices which invest in them.

The only reasonable motives for GPs to acquire computers are improvement of patient care, and relief of justifiable anxieties that if we do not, we are likely to lose touch with the future of clinical medicine. These motives are excellent, but they don't pay the mortgage.

Computers can perform entirely new and potentially valuable tasks that would be impossible — indeed could hardly be conceived of — without them; for example, listing all the patients with combined diabetes and hypertension, or revising criteria for diagnosis or treatment in an entire practice list in the light of new evidence. Using them to perform tasks that are now done manually, however, is rarely if ever economic. To the extent that all improvements in management efficiency tend to reveal omissions that might otherwise be conveniently overlooked, computers are likely not only to cost a lot of money, but also to increase medical workload.

As regards patient care, I still see no case for installing a computerised information system unless and until you have developed ordinary office methods, good A4 records, special box-files, lists and indexes of all kinds, to their fullest possible extent. Only when these possibilities are exhausted is it worth computerising the data; and at that point your data will at last be in a form suitable for the computer to receive.

The Glyncorrwg practice reached this point in 1984, and for the past year we have been laying the foundations for a new information system. We expect to spend at least a year with it before it replaces the manual systems we use for call and recall, and we are fairly sure that it will never replace manual records altogether. We have followed the advice of Dr Vince Cooper (1984), of Waterhouses in Cheshire, of avoiding all off-the-peg systems, and developing our own to our own requirements using a business database (Compsoft Delta 4) with a microcomputer powerful enough to have ample reserve capacity for our two populations of 1700 and 2000 (two Apricot PCs and a Plus Five 20 megabyte hard disc). Though this involves some expensive training for our practice manager, it allows us to develop our own ideas in our own way and to change our minds, as we certainly shall in the light of experience. It also means we are using business software which has already been in use on a mass scale for several years, completely debugged, which is certainly not the case with off-the-peg GP packages.

LEARNING COMPUTERS

The second reasonable motive for using computers, to avoid being left so far behind that you can never catch up, can be met without going to the expense of a fully developed information system. You can now get a word processor and printer for less than £500. This is immediately useful for the practice in doing letters, printing name and address labels, organising teaching material, and storing in an accessible and unlosable form the many bits and pieces of information hitherto buried under various forgotten piles at home, in the office, or somewhere in or on your consulting room desk. By the time you really need an information system, you and your staff will be handy with the keyboard and no longer afraid of computers.

The broad question of computers in general practice has been dealt with excellently in general terms by Lewis Ritchie (1984).

REFERENCES

Cooper V 1984 Third time lucky. Practice Computing 3:9

Hannay D R, Mitchell S 1985 Storing summary patient data as a microcomputer file. Journal of the Royal College of General Practitioners 35:525

Ritchie L D 1984 Computers in primary care: practicalities and prospects. William Heinemann Medical Books, London

Weed L L 1969 Medical records, medical education, and patient care. Case Western Reserve Press, Cleveland

10

Measurements

Figure 10.1 shows the association between the mean of three readings of phase V diastolic pressure and subsequent annual mortality, for men aged 35–44, free from organ damage at entry (Kannel & Gordon 1970). Case-finding and follow-up measurements aim to place individual patients accurately on this predictive curve, so that we can be sure that treatment is both worthwhile and effective in reducing pressure.

Because this graph presents not raw data as actually observed, but data smoothed to illustrate the underlying truth of the association between diastolic pressure and mortality, it eliminates both observer bias and digit preference in the diastolic readings. These can be seen very easily for diastolic, but not for systolic pressure, in Figure 10.2, derived from the raw data on which Figure 10.1

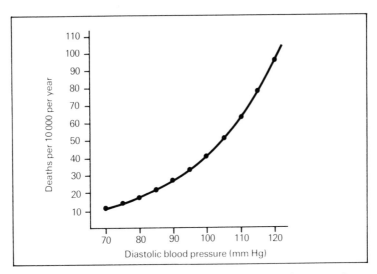

Fig. 10.1 Risk function for mortality against diastolic pressure in men aged 35–44 years (Kannel & Gordon 1970).

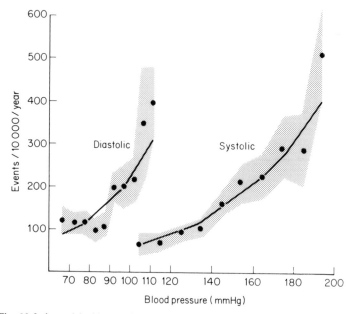

Fig. 10.2 Annual incidence of cardiovascular events at Framingham over 18 years of follow-up, by level of blood pressure in all ages, and with the means of male and female rates. Shaded areas indicate 95% confidence limits of individual data points, based on the assumption that the numbers of events behave as Poisson variables (Anderson 1978). (Reproduced with permission from *The Lancet*).

was based (Anderson 1978). There is no bias and less digit preference apparent for systolic pressures in Figure 10.2, presumably because the clinicians recording the pressures were used to a diastolic rather than a systolic classification of risk.

Other potential sources of error are shown in Figure 10.3 (Bevan et al 1969), showing pressures recorded at 5-min intervals from an intra-arterial catheter worn by a hypertensive subject over a 24-h period. The peak just before sleep is associated with coitus, an unlikely occasion for measurement of casual blood pressure in the GP's surgery, but not such an unlikely source of error; just thinking about it has a substantial effect.

Your hypertension control programme can be no better than the measurements on which it is based. Good quality data for personal care of individual patients are not less but more important than for epidemiological research on groups, but you would hardly think so from the way these measurements are usually made both in general practice and in hospitals.

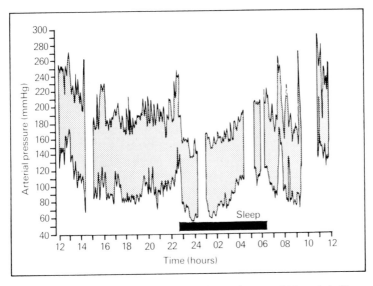

Fig. 10.3 Arterial pressure, plotted at 5-min intervals over a 24-h period. The period of sleep is shown by the horizontal bar. Patient x with essential hypertension in the benign phase (Bevan et al 1969).

SOURCES OF ERROR

Error in measurement means putting people on expensive, potentially uncomfortable and occasionally dangerous medication which they do not need, or (less frequently) ignoring blood pressures that are apparently safe but are in fact poorly controlled. There are three main sources of error: the patient, the observer, and the instrument.

The patient

However carefully conditions are standardised and patients put at their ease, attempts to characterise any patient's average pressure throughout the year by a single reading will obviously fail. It is true that in a group of patients, casual seated arterial pressure closely approximates to mean pressure as measured throughout the waking day by portable semi-continuous recorders for subjects not doing any heavy manual work or taking strenuous exercise (Sokolow et al 1966). It is also true that in the Framingham study, a single initial casual pressure reading was found to be almost as good a predictor of risk as the mean of several readings (Kannel & Sorlie 1975). But these are conclusions from grouped rather than individual data; the fact that the average male takes a size 8 shoe is not a reason for not making any other sizes.

Figure 10.4 shows what happened in Glyncorrwg (Hart 1974) when we repeated the readings on patients aged 20–64 who were found initially to have diastolic pressures high enough to require treatment on the criteria we were then using (men <40 years: diastolic blood pressure >100 mmHg; 40–64, >105; women <40, >115; 40–64, >110). The 97 found on the first screen fell to 47 after two readings, and 38 after three readings. A study of a large sample of practices in north-west London in 1982 (Kurji & Haines 1984) showed that almost half (46%) of all antihypertensive treatment was initiated after a single reading. Had I followed that course in Glyncorrwg, nearly three times as many people would have been started on treatment.

No patient should ever be started on antihypertensive drugs on the evidence of one reading. Even in the uncommon case of a true hypertensive emergency, it should be possible to record three replicate pressures, and even these often show a substantial fall as the alerting reflex subsides. Cases picked up by case-finding are not emergencies, even with very high pressures, providing retinal haemorrhage and oedema have been sought and not found. With these there is always time to repeat measurements at least three times on separate days, which also allows more time for all-round

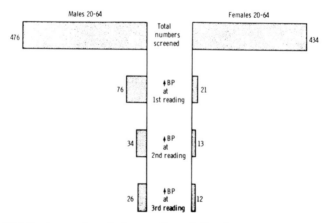

Fig. 10.4 Persistence through three readings of diastolic pressures classed as hypertensive. Glyncorrwg 1968, screened population (Hart 1974).

assessment, patient education, and the beginnings of a good contractual relationship.

When our nurses find a high pressure, they now arrange for the patient to return twice more for repeat readings, without any prompting from the GP. Even so, in many borderline cases we are uncertain whether to begin treatment. The alternatives are either to arrange for weekly readings by the practice nurse over a couple of months, or to teach patients to measure their own pressures and bring back the results.

Home readings

Using an electronic sphygmomanometer, almost any patient or relative can learn to measure blood pressure with about 5 minutes of teaching from a practice nurse. Asked to measure pressure twice a day for 2 weeks, virtually all do so.

Home readings by patients have been shown to agree well with hospital outpatient readings by doctors (Wilkinson & Raftery 1978). It is also true that mean pressures at home (measured by continuous intra-arterial readings by ambulatory monitoring) have been found to be higher (by 14 mmHg systolic pressure) than in the same patients admitted to a hospital ward, even when rest and activity in the two situations are taken into account (Young et al 1983). It seems reasonable to conclude that hospital outpatient conditions resemble those of the GP's surgery more closely than those of inpatients on a hospital ward.

From 28 home readings it is a simple matter to work out the mean with a pocket calculator and take a decision based on it.

Home readings are of great help in identifying hyper-reactors to office measurements, however carefully the *readings* are made. These people are a small minority, but the gap between mean office and home measurements can be remarkable. An example is shown in Figure 10.5. These people may still have an important problem. The Framingham data suggest that people with hyper-reactive pressures are at higher risk, of the same order as people whose high pressures are more stable, and that in any case, variability of blood pressure is not a stable characteristic (Kannell et al 1980). It is difficult to interpret this evidence in a practical way (unless you adopt the policy of just zapping every raised pressure with drugs, as soon as its head appears above the 90 mmHg skyline). Probably the best policy is simply to keep an eye on these people by annual blood pressure checks without treatment, a policy which patients

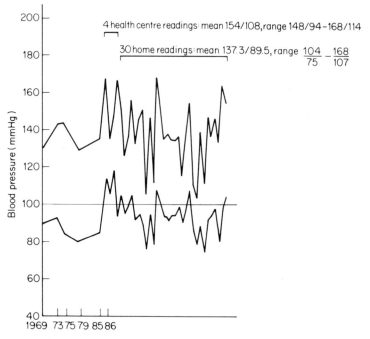

Fig. 10.5 Blood pressure readings at home and at the health centre for female patient SMJ, aged 33 in 1969.

seem to find intelligible and acceptable. Most of them eventually develop higher pressures needing treatment, often after many years of observation.

There is a valuable hidden agenda in this exercise. Patients are usually astonished at their own discovery of the variability of untreated pressure under reasonably constant home conditions. They can then begin to understand the probabilistic nature of human biology and rational medical care, the dangers of blind faith and the value of constructive scepticism.

Anxiety and fear

It goes almost without saying that it is a waste of time recording pressures in frightened or angry patients, but this is not always obvious. Untreated patients with normal or slow pulse rates are unlikely to be stressed in this way, and routine recording of pulse rates provides useful additional evidence for interpreting pressure values in individual cases. It is often helpful to ask patients whether they do feel anxiety, fear or anger when they come to the doctor. Many patients admit to these feelings when asked directly, and once this has been done, it often seems to be the first step in getting rid of them.

The effect of anxiety or even mere curiosity has been beautifully shown by studies in Milan, plotting continuous intra-arterial readings in 48 hypertensive and normotensive subjects lying in hospital beds (Mancia et al 1983). In nearly all cases pressures rose as doctors arrived at the bedside to measure blood pressure in the usual way, by a mean 27 mmHg systolic and 15 mmHg diastolic pressure over the previous resting intra-arterial value. There were big individual differences in the extent of this rise, with a range of 4–75 mmHg systolic and 1–36 mmHg diastolic pressure.

Though it is essential to bear this sort of evidence in mind, it is difficult to use it intelligently in practice. The evidence on which rational management policies are based is (fortunately for us) not from intra-arterial readings and ambulatory monitoring, but from casual seated blood pressures measured in much the same way as in ordinary general practice. The search for 'true' blood pressures, uncontaminated by response to the real world our patients live in, which so occupied the minds of pioneers such as Smirk in New Zealand, was probably futile. It has now been shown that basal pressures are no better correlated with organ damage than casual pressures (Caldwell et al 1978).

Cold

Chilling of the body raises blood pressure substantially, and this seems to account for systematic differences between pressures recorded in summer and winter, which are well known to epidemiologists (Hawthorne & Smalls 1980). Obviously, waiting rooms should be warm, but with an efficient appointments system this may not be much help on a cold winter evening. We have found that the only thing we can do about it is to remain aware of the problem; in a really cold winter, the proportion of hypertension clinic patients with poor control rises substantially.

Full bladders

This is a potent and often forgotten elevator of blood pressure. The minority of junior surgical staff who measure blood pressure routinely in emergency admissions frequently send for their physician colleagues to pronounce an opinion on old men with acute retention. These patients return home after prostatectomy with their original normal blood pressures plus an expensive and unnecessary array of antihypertensive drugs.

Full bladders also happen in full waiting rooms, with the same misleading effect. The man who stopped off for a quick pint on the way to the surgery suddenly realises that if he goes to the toilet he may lose his place in the queue. He grits his teeth, clenches his sphincters, and raises his diastolic pressure by 20 or 30 mmHg. As Charcot said, listen to the patient and he will tell you the diagnosis.

Circadian rhythm?

There have been bitter arguments about whether there is, or is not, a systematic difference between morning and evening blood pressures. Blood pressure falls dramatically during sleep, as a rule even in malignant hypertension. There is good evidence of a substantial rise just before waking and for an hour or two after, but a huge US study of 10 000 men and women aged 30–64 showed no significant difference between systolic or diastolic pressures measured in the morning and the afternoon (Mayer et al 1978).

The observer

The observer can influence pressure through his or her effect on the patient; by inspiring fear, love, loathing, and doubtless other passions, but perhaps most often simply irritation. All of these can modify pressure, and may account for the systematic differences between pressures recorded by nurses and by doctors, which are discussed in Chapter 11.

Observers influence measurements in three other important ways; digit preference, bias, and by their attitude to the results.

Digit preference

Digit preference is the name applied to a clinical fact, that when asked to mark a uniformly descending target against a vertical scale of measurement marked at 2 mm intervals with un-numbered lines, and at 5 mm intervals with terminal 5s and 0s, observers prefer 0s. Those who consistently read 0s are clearly reading to the nearest 10 mmHg. Whether they choose the nearest 10 up or the nearest

10 down is not known; perhaps there are optimists and pessimists. Either way, this seems a casual way to make a measurement used for making important clinical decisions.

Is this kind of shooting from the hip common in otherwise good clinicians? Table 10.1 shows some evidence from hospital correspondence containing a total of 39 readings concerning 5 randomly sampled patients from the Glyncorrwg practice. For comparison, 110 readings by our practice nurses for the same patients over the same period are given. Clearly, 10% of the readings should end in 0 and another 10% in 5.

Table 10.1 Percentages of various terminal digits in blood pressure readings

	Hospital medical staff		Glyncorrwg practice doctors and nurses	
	n	%	n	%
Systolic				
Terminal 0	37	95	27	24
Terminal 5	2	5	2	2
Terminal other	0	0	81	74
Diastolic				
Terminal 0	33	85	20	18
Terminal 5	6	15	4	4
Terminal other	0	0	86	78
Total readings	39	100	110	100

These data include readings from a university department of cardiology. If you have a look at your own records you will probably find much the same monotonous preference for zeros, but as you see, you are in good company.

Bias

Bias is the tendency of observers unconsciously to 'make sense' of measurements by allocating them unambiguously to one side or the other of a cutting point habitually used for clinical decision. If you return to Figure 10.2 you will see a relatively even distribution of systolic pressure values over the range 105–175 mmHg, with an unexpected dip at 185 and a rise at 195 which could be partly explained by smaller numbers and therefore greater sampling error. There is little evidence of bias, because in the early 1960s, when these data were collected, systolic pressures were virtually ignored in clinical decision-making. If you look at the diastolic pressures, on the other hand, there is a clear break exactly where you would expect to find it, if the population were neatly divided into normotensives up to and including 90 mmHg, and hypertensives over 90 mmHg. Indeed, the values are distributed as a three-step staircase rather than a curve; normotensives, mild hypertensives, and severe hypertensives.

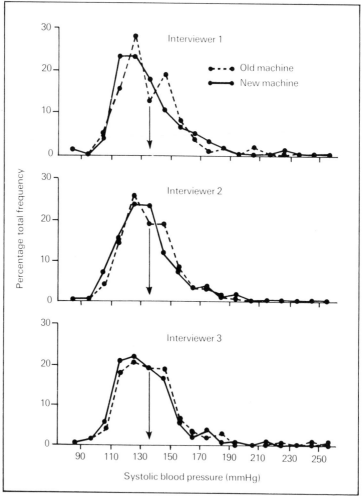

Fig. 10.6 Frequency distributions of readings of systolic pressure by different observers in the same population, using standard and random-zero sphygmomanometers (Humerfelt 1966).

Is this a slander on the certainly honest and conscientious group of experienced observers who set up the early years of the Framingham study? Not at all; this is how all clinicians behaved, until made aware of this universal tendency. Figure 10.6 shows a study comparing readings by Norwegian cardiovascular epidemiologists with a thoroughly clinical background, using conventional sphygmomanometers (as used in the entry phase of the Framingham study), and also a random-zero sphygmomanometer, which allows observers to make a reading without knowing its value, and is therefore bias-free (Humerfelt 1966). The illustration shows systolic values rather than diastolic, but as continental European doctors paid a lot more attention to systolic pressures than Anglo-Americans, the effect is obvious; a cleavage at systolic 140 mmHg, apparent with conventional sphygmomanometers, disappears with unbiased readings.

Bias is important in two situations; initial grouping of a screened population, and follow-up of treated cases. Publications comparing different antihypertensive treatments or auditing clinical managements are of questionable value if they are based on conventional sphygmomanometers. The best but very expensive solution to this problem is to use a Hawksley random-zero sphygmomanometer for all measurements. This has been our policy in Glyncorrwg; since 1974 all office readings have been made in this way. The cheaper and more practical solution is to use electronic sphygmomanometers. These have some serious limitations, discussed later in this chapter, but they are wonderful for teaching unbiased measurement technique, which can be learned. Fully retrained observers, who have become conscious of this universal trait, can use conventional sphygmomanometers without bias.

Attitudes to measurement

This pedantry may be all very well for epidemiological research, but does it really matter for day-to-day clinical medicine? Do the statements 'BP 120/70' or '170/100' reveal an experienced clinician, aware of the fallibility of these measurements and careful to avoid the spurious precision implied by the statements 'BP 124/68' or '166/102'? To hit so erratic a target as hypertension, isn't a shotgun better than a precision rifle?

The analogy is a good one. If the search for hypertension is run like a pheasant shoot, in which the objective is to kill as many birds and as few beaters as possible, then all you can do is to classify targets as either in the air or on the ground, minimising errors by not shooting close to the skyline; but control of hypertension in a general practice population is not a one-off blitz, but a sustained search for precise targets, with many opportunities for collecting the evidence necessary for accurate decisions. Surely this evidence, on which a decision whether or not to intervene must at some point be taken, should be of the highest possible quality?

The instrument

There are basically four types of sphygmomanometer available; aneroid, conventional mercury, research, and electronic. All of them have one thing in common, an inflatable cuff. This is the most serious source of error arising from the instrument itself.

Cuffs

Unless the rubber bag inside the cuff reaches about two-thirds of the way round the arm, with the centre of the bag placed accurately over the brachial artery, a serious false-high error may be introduced in the readings. For adults, a cuff-width at or over 11 cm seems to be all right for almost any arm, but cuff length is critical (Croft 1982; King 1982). One study showed that in readings taken with a rubber bag which did not encircle the arm, there was an average systolic error of 23 and a diastolic error of 19 mmHg (Orma et al 1960). If the cuff is applied with care, such a criterion may be too stringent, but other studies have shown that 82% of adult British arms are too big for our standard 23 cm cuff, and 50% of US arms are too big for their standard 26 cm cuff (Conceicao et al 1976). The effect is purely artefactual, and has nothing to do with the true association of hypertension with obesity.

In 1983 a woman of 47 moved into my practice; she had been taking various antihypertensive drugs continuously for the previous 18 years. She had been started on treatment at age 29 after a single reading of 145/100 mmHg, presumably using a standard cuff. She was 5ft 1 in (1.51 m) tall and weighed 14 st 2 lb (89.9 kg), giving a body mass index of 39.4. Her previous GP record showed the readings given in Table 10.2.

The answer is, of course, to get outsize cuffs and use them. This is no longer as difficult as it was; both Accoson and Baumanometer, the chief suppliers, now make a full range of cuff sizes, though you often have to be very persistent to obtain them. Both brands use

Table 10.2 Blood pressure readings of a 47-year-old woman as noted on her GP record

Age (years)	BP (mmHg)	Events
29	145/100	Started Rx
	130/80	
	130/80	
37	160/90	
43	190/100	
45	170/105	
	170/105	
	160/96	
	170/96	
47	162/100	
	with a standard cuff,	
	falling to	
	142/80	
	with an outsize cuff.	
		Rx stopped.
		'Hypertension' cured.

a system of transverse lines (easier to use than to describe) which give an immediately obvious indication of whether you are using the right cuff. As most arms are 'outsize' we normally use the 'large adult' as standard, occasionally replacing it with the 'normal adult' or 'very large adult' when we need to. Using too long a cuff introduces no error.

Most cuffs now use Velcro binding, which is deceptively convenient. It makes the bag too rigid, and after a few years the nylon hooklets lose their grip and begin to slip unless they are cleaned by vigorous scrubbing with a nylon toothbrush. Plain cloth cuffs, with a tuck-in at the end, are better.

Aneroid sphygmomanometers

Aneroid sphygmomanometers are compact — otherwise there is nothing to commend them. Fisher (1978) compared over 3000 aneroid machines in use with a standard mercury manometer and found an error of more than 7 mmHg in 10% of them. The dial is small so that precise readings are difficult over the very compressed scale available. If anything begins to go wrong, measurements drift up or down imperceptibly, producing a systematic error over all readings which may go on for months or years before it is suspected. Aneroid sphygmomanometers require adjustment above sea level, which they rarely receive, and errors increase at higher levels of blood pressure.

Mercury sphygmomanometers

Mercury sphygmomanometers are cumbersome, particularly for home visits, and need maintenance which they rarely get, but they have the great advantages of simplicity, and when they break down the error is usually obvious to observers unless they take their equipment wholly for granted. Details of maintenance are given in Appendix II, which can be photocopied for use by practice staff responsible.

Spot checks of hospital sphymomanometers in regular use generally show about half of them to be seriously faulty (Conceicao et al 1976; Burke et al 1982), because of a long medical and nursing tradition that all instruments live until they die, without care, testing, or maintenance. One of the pharmaceutical companies (Riker Laboratories) offers a free sphygmomanometer maintenance service for GPs.

Research sphygmomanometers

The greatest research need is for a non-invasive, portable sphygmomanometer which will give semi-continuous readings over about 24 hours, and permit the subject under study to lead a normal home and working life; an instrument with much the same qualities as a portable ECG monitor. Despite some claims to the contrary, at the time of writing (1986) no such instrument exists.

The standard research instrument remains the cumbersome, expensive, but reliable and easily maintained random-zero machine (Wright & Dore 1970) marketed by Hawksley, and familiar in many British practices because of its use in the MRC trial.

Electronic sphygmomanometers

The potential advantages of electronic sphygmomanometers are so great that they are bound eventually to replace mercury machines in most circumstances. They eliminate digit preference and bias, and with a fixed deflation rate can eliminate rapid descent as a major source of error. These qualities taken together virtually eliminate differences between observers (including patients as their own observers), except for different emotional effects on the patient.

They are generally easy to use, and are therefore particularly suitable for home readings.

Despite these potential advantages, their general use now cannot yet be recommended. Thorough evaluation of the electronic machines available in the 1970s at the start of the HDFP trial revealed none that were better or more reliable than the random-zero machine, and the designers of the later MRC trial seem to have reached the same conclusion. There are still problems about reliability and cuff size.

One problem with electronic machines is that if they begin to go wrong this may not be apparent to the user, and a systematic error may be introduced which may go uncorrected for years. If a mercury machine goes wrong it is usually obvious, and the machine can be cleaned and repaired on the spot; if an electronic machine goes wrong, the error will probably be silent and certainly be incomprehensible. Makers' literature is always inadequate, often transliterated from Japanese, and rarely contains anything about possible faults, not even so simple or frequent a matter as the effect of a dying battery. Both salesmen and many purchasers seem to have such faith in all things electronic that any differences between readings obtained with a mercury and an electronic machine are automatically attributed to faults in the traditional equipment, though nearly always the reverse is the case.

The cheaper machines rely on a microphone in the cuff which picks up an acoustic signal from the brachial artery, just as your ear does through the stethoscope. Accurate placement over the artery is even more important than with a mercury machine. The more expensive ones operate from a very sensitive pressure transducer programmed to distinguish a pulse wave from other extraneous signals, a big step forward which may eliminate many possible sources of error.

Unfortunately both types complicate the cuff problem. I know of only one make, the Phillips machine, that is able to supply an outsize cuff on request. This is not big enough for really large arms, but will cope with most if used as standard. This is the one we have used for our home readings, but we have had a lot of trouble with it, particularly with diastolic pressures, and have now reverted to a standard mercury machine.

We must hope that one day the British Standards Institution or the Consumers' Association will test these various electronic machines, telling us how many of them have meaningfully different concealed insides, as opposed to visible (and therefore saleable) outsides, encouraging the more responsible suppliers to improve their products and assisting the early demise of some of the outwardly impressive rubbish on the market.

DIASTOLIC PHASES IV AND V

Until the early 1970s, most British doctors were taught to use phase IV (muffling of the Korotkoff sounds) as a diastolic endpoint, and American doctors were taught to use phase V (disappearance of sound). There followed a period of uncertainty, from which doctors on both sides of the Atlantic seem now to be groping toward consensus agreement on phase V.

Two sets of arguments have been deployed for and against these alternatives. First there are arguments about which most nearly approximates to intra-arterial diastolic pressure. The evidence from various studies is conflicting, but phase IV seems to average about 8, and phase V about 2 mmHg above intra-arterial diastolic pressure. Secondly, and I think more importantly, phase V is much easier to recognise and therefore for nurses (who will actually make most of the readings) to use. Doctors have been found to show twice as much variability in recording diastolic as systolic pressures, and nurses three times as much (Richardson & Robinson 1971).

Though phase V should be standard practice, there are patients in whom sounds never completely disappear down to 0 mmHg, even with all clothing removed from the upper arm. There is then no alternative to using phase IV. When this happens the fact should be noted. The conventional correction is to subtract 5 mmHg for equivalent phase V diastolic pressure, but the gap between phases IV and V is extremely variable, from almost nothing to about 10 mmHg, and the average difference is probably around 8 mmHg (D'Souza & Irwig 1976).

SYSTOLIC AND DIASTOLIC PRESSURES

One simple way of avoiding all the ambiguities of diastolic pressure is to pay more attention to systolic pressure, and all the evidence favours this course. In both men and women over the age of 40, systolic pressures are better predictors of subsequent cardiovascular disease than diastolic pressures at all ages and all levels of pressure (Kannel et al 1971). Enlargement of the heart (Kannel et al 1969), heart failure (Kannel et al 1972), ischaemic heart disease, stroke

(Kannel et al 1970) and ECG response to antihypertensive treatment (George et al 1972; Ibrahim et al 1977) are all more closely related to systolic than to diastolic pressures attained.

Unfortunately we have all learned to speak diastolic language, and in practice doctors avoid taking clinical decisions along two scales rather than one. Though all innovating clinicians have known the superiority of systolic over diastolic measurements for many years, we continue to speak and write diastolese for fear of being ignored or misunderstood. Diastolic pressures therefore continue to be used as thresholds both for entry to treatment and for assessment of control. This has serious consequences, particularly for older patients. Very high systolic pressures, say over 200 mmHg, are frequently ignored in both initial assessment and follow-up, if the diastolic pressure is reassuringly low, as it frequently is. This is legitimised by the myth of systolic hypertension as a normal accompaniment of old age, which 'only reflects the state of the peripheral arteries' (I quote from a recent professorial statement). As the state of peripheral arteries, including those supplying the heart and brain, are our principal concern in treating high blood pressure, the logic of this argument escapes me. I have tried to translate more of this edition into systolese, but it's a long battle.

REFERENCES

Anderson T W 1978 Re-examination of some of the Framingham blood pressure data. Lancet ii:1139
Bevan A T, Honour A J, Stott F H et al 1969 Direct arterial pressure recording in unrestricted man. Clinical Science 36:329
Burke M J, Towers H M, O'Malley K, Fitzgerald D J, O'Brien E T 1982 Sphygmomanometers in hospital and family practice: problems and recommendations. British Medical Journal 285:469
Caldwell J R, Schork M A, Aiken R D 1978 Is near basal blood pressure a more accurate predictor of cardiorenal manifestations of hypertension than casual blood pressure? Journal of Chronic Diseases 31:507
Conceicao S, Ward M K, Kerr D N S 1976 Defects in sphygmomanometers: an important source of error in blood pressure recording. British Medical Journal 1:886
Croft P R 1982 Sphygmomanometer cuff sizes. Lancet ii:323
D'Souza M F, Irwig L M 1976 Measurement of blood pressure. British Medical Journal iv:814
Fisher H W 1978 Cardiovascular Medicine 3:769 quoted by Paul O 1979 Clinical aspects of the natural history of mild hypertension. In: Gross F, Strasser T (eds) Mild hypertension: natural history and management. Pitman Medical, London, p 15
George C F, Breckenridge A M, Dollery C T 1972 Value of routine electrocardiography in hypertensive patients. British Heart Journal 34:618

Hart J T 1974 The marriage of primary care and epidemiology. Journal of the Royal College of Physicians of London 8:299

Hawthorne V M, Smalls M 1980 Blood pressure and ambient temperature. British Medical Journal 280:567

Humerfelt S 1966 Methodology of blood pressure recording. In: Gross F (ed) Antihypertensive therapy. Springer Verlag, Berlin

Ibrahim M M, Tarazi, R C, Dustan H P et al 1971 Electrocardiogram in evaluation of resistance to antihypertensive therapy. Archives of Internal Medicine 137:1125

Kannel W B, Gordon T 1970 The Framingham study: an epidemiological investigation of cardiovascular disease, section 26. Government Printing Office, Washington DC

Kannel W B, Sorlie P 1975 Hypertension in Framingham. In: Paul O (ed) Epidemiology and control of hypertension. Stratton Intercontinental Medical Book, New York, p 553

Kannel W B, Gordon T, Offutt D 1969 Left ventricular hypertrophy by electrocardiogram: prevalence, incidence, and mortality in the Framingham study. Annals of Internal Medicine 71:89

Kannel W B, Wolf, Verter J et al 1970 Epidemiologic assessment of the role of blood pressure in stroke. Journal of the American Medical Association 214:301

Kannel W B, Castelli W P, McNamara P M et al 1972 Role of blood pressure in the development of congestive heart failure. New England Journal of Medicine 287:782

Kannel W B, Gordon T, Schwartz M J 1971 Systolic versus diastolic blood pressure and risk of coronary heart disease: the Framingham study. American Journal of Cardiology 27:335

Kannel W B, Sorlie T, Gordon T 1980 Labile hypertension: a faulty concept? Circulation 61:1183

King G E 1982 Selection of blood pressure cuff design. Lancet ii:492

Kurji K H, Haines A P 1984 Detection and management of hypertension in general practices in north-west London. British Medical Journal 288:903

Mancia G, Bertinieri G, Grassi G et al 1983 Effects of blood pressure measurement by the doctor on patients' blood pressure and heart rate. Lancet ii:695

Mayer K, Stamler J, Dyer A R et al 1978 Epidemiologic findings on the relationship of time of day and time since last meal to five clinical variables: serum cholesterol, hematocrit, systolic and diastolic pressure, and heart rate. Preventive Medicine 7:22

Orma E, Punsar S, Karvonen M 1960 Mansetti hypertonia. Duodecim 76:460

Richardson J F, Robinson D 1971 Variations in the measurement of blood pressure between doctors and nurses. Journal of the Royal College of General Practitioners 21:698

Sokolow M, Werdegar D, Kain H K et al 1966 Relationship between level of blood pressure measured casually and by portable recorders and severity of complications in essential hypertension. Circulation 34:279

Wilkinson P R, Raftery E B 1978 Patient attitudes to measuring their own blood pressure. British Medical Journal ii:824

Wright B M, Dore C F 1970 A random-zero sphygmomanometer. Lancet i:337

Young M A, Rowlands D B, Stallard T J et al 1983 Effect of environment on blood pressure: home versus hospital. British Medical Journal 286:1235

11

Divisions of labour

Any practice which undertakes full ascertainment and control of high blood pressure for its whole population, even if it restricts medication to the 5–10% of adults with pressures >175/105 mmHg or hypertensive organ damage, invites workload far beyond the capacity of GPs working alone. Even with a full complement of employed and attached staff, all hands are on deck. Divisions of labour and responsibility are essential, and need planning from the outset.

WHO DOES WHAT?

It is usually taken for granted that all work should be delegated so far as possible downward, so that the most skilled people do the most skilled work. GPs who automatically regard themselves as more skilled and more valuable than anyone else in the team will quickly find they no longer have one.

The most effective approach is for the whole team to consider thoroughly and in detail what has to be done, and who there is to do it. Then responsibilities should be allocated by agreement, on a trial basis subject to revision at later meeting, when new decisions can be taken in the light of audit and experience.

One of the first questions is who will do the blood pressure readings. Granted a short period of appropriate retraining, nurses measure pressures more accurately, with fewer preconceptions, and cause less alarm to patients than doctors. Figures 11.1 and 11.2 show the distributions of systolic and diastolic pressures measured by nurses and doctors on the same group of patients. Nurse-measured pressures are consistently lower than doctor-measured pressures, particularly in the high systolic range.

Other tasks undertaken by nurses in Glyncorrwg are checking medication (using the tablets patients are asked to bring with them always); decisions to organise repeat blood pressure measurements;

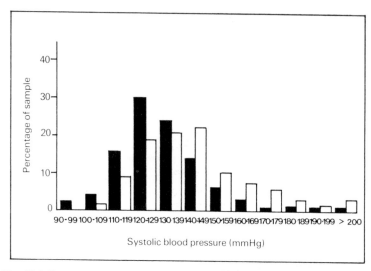

Fig. 11.1 Frequency distribution of systolic blood pressures measured by nurses (■) and by doctors (□) (Richardson & Robinson 1971).

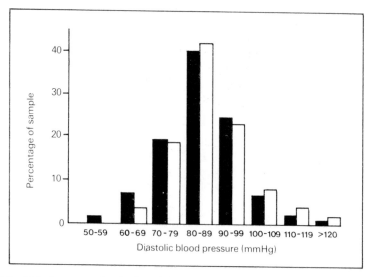

Fig. 11.2 Frequency distribution of diastolic blood pressures measured by nurses (■) and by doctors (□) (Richardson & Robinson 1971).

weighing; height measurements; pulse rates; measurement of haemoglobin; all venous blood sampling; centrifuging and preparation of blood slides; urine testing (tapes and dip-cultures); measurement of peak expiratory flow rates, and ECG recording.

Tasks undertaken by the doctor but not the nurse are integration of hypertension management with management of other problems; search for specific side-effects, such as lethargy, depression, diminished libido and impotence; updating of alcohol histories; examination of fundi through dilated pupils in patients whose pressures are out of control (otherwise we don't check fundi routinely); of the chest and heart for crackles, valvular disease, and arrhythmias; and of the legs for oedema and absent pulses; and all decisions about starting, stopping, or changing antihypertensive medication and institution of laboratory and radiological investigations.

Completion of laboratory and X-ray request forms is done by doctors and not delegated to nurses, because we think they already have quite enough unskilled, tedious and repetitive work to do. Computer-generated name and address labels are now a great help; we keep a full sheet of these inside each record folder, and print a new one when they are used up.

Tasks shared by both doctor and nurse are friendly chat and general enquiries about health and worries, updating of smoking history, and responsibility for chasing up defaulters.

These divisions of labour have gradually evolved over many years, and should continue to change. They partly depend on the aptitude, interests, and often the family responsibilities and other pressures on time of the nurse, and of the doctor. The idea that divisions of labour can be set for all time by higher administrations is one of the most damaging effects of the present hierarchical structure of community nursing, which must change if we are to achieve integration of general practice and community nursing.

RESPONSIBILITIES FOR MANAGEMENT AND LEADERSHIP

Doctors have a long period of training in which they are stuffed with technical knowledge originally acquired by scientific techniques, but they are not trained in scientific methods of sceptical experiment. Once they have tenure and no longer face the examiners, only a minority of doctors (a large minority, it's true), either in hospital or general practice, continue to follow the serious literature and to innovate, applying scientific advances to the particular circumstances of their own populations. All good GPs are specialists — specialists in their own patch with its own people; Glyncorrwgologists, Blaengwynfologists, Bollingtologists, Lowereastsidologists, or whatever. If they accept this, they are normally better equipped to initiate new work than anyone else in the team. Having initiated it, almost anyone — doctors, nurses, office staff — may develop a leading role, and in any case, with time, a team working correctly becomes a collective within which people are able to work autonomously, each pushing forward his or her own frontier but in a commonly agreed general direction. The key to this process is acceptance of measurable objectives, with regular audit of the extent to which they are being achieved; authority must be based on evidence rather than status.

Often senior doctors don't accept responsibility for leading this work, and the question then arises whether anyone else can. Junior doctors may have sufficient diplomatic skill to push their seniors aside into the role of constitutional monarchs, and nurses or practice managers may occasionally get grudging agreement to be allowed to pursue their own mad schemes, as long as they don't disturb anyone else. The trouble is, they nearly always do. Changing to another practice is one solution, but not a helpful one for the patients.

USES OF AUDIT

Some practices are good at talking and others are not, but the number of practice meetings, and the hot air released in them, bear little relation to progress in patient care.

The most effective method for securing real change in any practice is to present a problem in quantified clinical terms which compel respect from doctors, nurses and office staff alike, to set modest objectives by consensus agreement and then follow up by measuring attainment of these objectives. The person with ideas can draw out a random sample of 25 records for people aged between 40 and 64 and spend three evenings evaluating the recording of information about blood pressure, smoking, and weight for height; or 25 known hypertensives, to see how many have been seen and checked within the last 4 months, how many contain a clear account of current medication, and how many were started on medication on reasonable criteria; or 25 known diabetics, to see how many have been reviewed in the past year, how many have had their fundi examined with pupils dilated, how many have blood pressures recorded and controlled, and how many have smoking status recorded.

Once targets are agreed (and if they are realistically modest, they will be difficult for even the most conservative doctor, nurse or office staff to resist), the rest follows. Once begun, the sequence

internally agreed target → internal verification → new internally agreed target

is usually unstoppable, providing targets are realistic and take fully into account the capacities and interests of the staff available.

THE EMPLOYED TEAM

Under the terms of the 1966 package deal, every GP principal is entitled to employ two whole-time equivalent (WTE) nursing or office staff, with 70% of wages reimbursed. Allowing for tax relief on the remaining 30% of wages, an employed practice nurse pays for herself if she does just two extra cervical smears a week for the practice for women in the qualifying age-group. However, in England and Wales the average number of ancillary staff employed by GPs has stuck at 1.1 for many years; 15 000 new people could be added to the primary care work force next week, if all GPs were to avail themselves fully of this facility.

Why don't they? Part of it is no doubt the still widespread belief that if you count the pennies, the pounds will look after themselves — a mean and squalid philosophy for what should be the most rapidly expanding sector in the NHS. Linked with this, but perhaps more important, is a more general fear of moving away from a small, idiosyncratic demand-led corner shop, to a large, collective organisation with big social responsibilities. Now that many more practice managers are coming into production, and structural changes in the GP service may be on the way, the picture could change rapidly; Robin Fraser's studies (Fraser & Gosling 1985a, 1985b, 1985c) of the attitudes of East Midlands GPs to assisted audit are a heartening indication of what may be possible. The Cumberlege report (DHSS 1986), despite its dismissive attitude to GPs employing practice nurses, opens up exciting possibilities for integration of general practice with community nursing, which if implemented by a future government could accelerate all the processes advocated in this book.

THE ATTACHED TEAM

Excellent work is being done in some prevention-oriented practices by community nurses attached to them with a specific remit to assist in hypertension control, in areas such as Oxford, with imaginative leadership from community physicians and nursing offices willing to commit real resources (Fullard et al 1984).

Unfortunately this is not typical. Where community nurses have been attached there is often a failure to integrate them properly in the team, so that they share fully in decision making, target setting and audit. Many GPs apparently still delegate work, but having done so, wash their hands of all further responsibility.

Here is a real example of blood pressure readings recorded by district nurses on a man who first presented with a left hemiplegia at the age of 66, was started on antihypertensive treatment with methyldopa 250 mg three times a day, and was handed over to the attached district nurses for monthly follow-up in 1977:

162/98	250/120→	200/130
180/90	240/110	220/130
190/110	180/120	200/130
220/120	200/130	180/110
220/120	200/130	190/110
230/120	180/90	170/100
180/120	180/100	180/120
220/150	190/130	180/120
220/140	200/130	180/110
230/140	190/110	170/100
180/140	190/130	210/110
120/100	198/134	temporarily moved home, entered new
190/100 →	250/150	practice, bendrofluazide added
		182/88
		154/80
		146/78
		150/69
		118/64
		moved back to original practice

This horrifying story was the result of delegating work without delegation of responsibility. It can happen all too easily if attachment is so loose that the community nurses are not really a part of the team.

Where health authorities are prepared to attach community nurses for this work, they must encourage continuity of staffing, so that the nurse can be trained on the job and really know the patients; and they must allow reasonable flexibility in job definition, so that the nurse can work both in a centre and in home follows-ups, and be allowed sufficient time for organisation and maintenance of records. Our experience in Glyncorrwg in both these respects has not been happy, and though there are honourable exceptions, at the time of writing (1986) this seems to be fairly general. The unfortunate result is that keen practices tend to employ their own nurses, so that bureaucracy is evaded rather than reformed.

Though there has been some discussion of a possible role for health visitors in preventive work among the middle-aged, this is hopelessly unrealistic unless there is a huge expansion of the health visitor work force, as well as a radical redefinition of their responsibilities. Health visitors seconded to work in this specific field, without responsibilities for children or the elderly, would be a different matter. Few health authorities seem as yet to have faced up to the implications for workload of translating preventive rhetoric into preventive action.

THE EXPANDED TEAM

Even in a GP hypertension clinic with a doctor and a nurse, it is difficult to do justice to control of other risk factors, particularly smoking, obesity, and reduced-fat diet. Everything depends on patient education, but that takes a lot of time, and needs reinforcement with specific literature which is often better, and certainly better received, if it is locally produced.

There is a great unmet need for mature, intelligent, honest, friendly, but not overprofessionalised women and men who could take responsibility for individual and group health education, for developing and making readily available short leaflets covering the specific things patients need to know and remember, in terms that link up with common local experience. Great numbers of just such people are now rotting in unemployment, but would certainly apply for such jobs if they were offered.

TRAINING

Training programmes are now an urgent need, for nurses and practice managers who are moving into this field, for attached community nurses, and hopefully for the lay counsellors described in the last paragraph. The few national meetings for these groups have been well supported, and there is no doubt that even now there is a large unsatisfied demand. Pharmaceutical companies, which in the absence of DHSS initiative remain responsible for meeting most of the cost of GP postgraduate education other than vocational training, are beginning to include nurses and other practice staff in their invitations. Ignorant hostility to the proposal of Council of the Royal College of General Practitioners for associate membership for non-medical practice staffs has set things back a little, but progress toward genuine inclusion of the whole team in continuing education will continue.

There remains a serious lack of locally organised courses, which could not only give training, but would also serve as forums for discussion among people trying to do the same job in different places, and devising their own solutions. This should be a top priority for District Health Authorities, or better still Primary Care Committees, if these were to replace Family Practitioner Committees as the Royal College of Nursing has suggested.

There is also a shortage of trainers. Practical preventive work cannot be taught effectively by people without experience of doing it, so this shortage will continue until we have a first generation of doctors and (particularly) nurses who have already achieved enough to give them the confidence and credibility to teach others. It is particularly important that whatever training courses are set up should not be weighed down with experts, but be conducted in a participative, small-group style, discussing real and representative data brought from the practices of the participants.

REFERENCES

Department of Health and Social Security 1986 Neighbourhood nursing: a focus for care (Cumberlege report). HMSO, London

Fraser R C, Gosling J T L 1985a Information systems for general practitioners for quality assessment: I. Responses of the doctors. British Medical Journal 291:1473

Fraser R C, Gosling J T L 1985b Information systems for general practitioners for quality assessment: II. Information preferences of the doctors. British Medical Journal 291:1444

Fraser R C, Gosling J T L 1985c Information systems for general practitioners for quality assessment: III. Suggested new prescribing profile. British Medical Journal 291:1613

Fullard E, Fowler G, Gray M 1984 Facilitating prevention in primary care. British Medical Journal 289:1585

Richardson J F, Robinson D 1971 Variations in the measurement of blood pressure between doctors and nurses. Journal of the Royal College of General Practitioners 21:698

12

Investigation, search for secondary hypertension and referral

Your hypertensives are identified, chiefly by organised search and occasionally by presenting symptoms, but always through measurement of a single variable — the blood pressure itself.

According to classical teaching, which for all I know may still continue in some medical schools, the next steps are firstly to verify that high pressure is sustained, secondly to search for causes, and finally to assess organ damage. For a referred outpatient, the first of these is likely to be completed by replicate readings at the first interview, and the other two will usually be completed in three interviews, at the end of which the patient will embark on a lifetime of treatment. Twenty minutes to half an hour will normally be available for these initial encounters, with help available for measurements, blood sampling, and form-filling.

In general practice, the time available for each interview is usually about 5 minutes' face-to-face time with the doctor. In Glyncorrwg we have managed to extend doctor-time to 10 minutes, plus about 5–10 minutes of nurse-time. There is no way we can do all that needs to be done in the first or even in the first three encounters, so we extend both verification and the collection of data over six or seven encounters, doing a little each time, and using each opportunity to convey information to the patient in small and hopefully memorable earfuls. A suggested sequence for this data collection is given at the end of this chapter.

VERIFICATION

There can be few more reckless gambles in clinical medicine than starting a patient on a lifetime of antihypertensive drugs on the evidence of a single reading, but on the evidence of records from 71 GPs who permitted audit of their records in 1976, this is what happened in about one-third of cases (Parkin et al 1979). The proportion of subjects with high pressure (using any threshold) falls by about half on second readings (on separate days), and by about 20% on the third reading. After this it is fairly stable, but there is still a large minority of patients whose blood pressures fall substantially over 3 or 4 months on observation alone.

In a well organised practice few patients are seen for whom antihypertensive treatment is so urgent that they would not benefit from a delay of a few weeks or even months, during which a full assessment can be made, uncontaminated by the effects of drugs. Even for the tiny minority who have a neuroretinopathy or heart failure when first seen, it is still possible to record at least three replicate readings spaced over 20 minutes or so. The fact that these often differ by 20 mmHg or more may be important evidence later on in assessing the apparent effects of antihypertensive drugs.

The routine in Glynccorwg is that when any pressure at or over a threshold of 170/100 mmHg is recorded, the nurses initiate another two visits to give us three readings to consider at the next doctor-consultation. About half our newly discovered hypertensives (mostly those with erratic readings or close to our borderline of 170/100 mmHg) borrow an electronic machine to record 14 days of morning and evening readings, so that the decisions to treat or not can be taken on the mean of 28 readings.

WHAT ABOUT OTHER RISK FACTORS?

Two other principal cardiovascular risk factors should be checked in everyone found to have a high pressure, whether or not you decide to start antihypertensive treatment: namely, smoking and blood cholesterol. Smoking status should always be checked at the same time as blood pressure, as a normal part of the same standard procedure. This helps to link the two risks in the minds of both patients and staff, and to emphasise the futility of treating hypertension while continuing to ignore smoking.

Many authorities deny the value of routine measurement of blood lipids in hypertensives, presumably on grounds of cost. This is trivial compared with the cost of much antihypertensive medication. Although there is a positive association between blood total cholesterol and obesity, and weight reduction is the first target in all cholesterol-lowering diets, there are plenty of skinny people with prodigiously high cholesterols; obesity is not a reliable indicator of cholesterol status. After many years of avoiding it (because it entails even more work for an already overworked team), I have been driven by the weight of evidence to the conclusion that action should be taken to reduce not only unusually high cholesterol values (say >7.5 mmol/dl), but all values more than about 5 mmol (about 200 mg)/dl in patients with one other major risk factor.

If such action is to be effective, it requires measurement, not guesswork. If we take trouble, so do our patients.

FAMILY HISTORY

Every patient should be asked about stroke, heart attacks and diabetes in parents and sibs; their smoking habits, and anything known about their blood pressure, though such information is seldom reliable. This is important partly in order to assess risk, but chiefly to develop motivation. Illness in the family is potentially the most valuable experience patients can have to help them to make rational decisions about their own lives. We put this information at the top of the summary sheet, so it is always readily available.

HISTORY, EXAMINATION AND BASELINE MEASUREMENTS

Starting antihypertensive drug treatment without taking a directed history and without a physical examination of any kind is still common. At the stage when most of them are picked up in a well organised general practice, few hypertensives have gross evidence of organ damage. Routine physical examination therefore may seem a pointless exercise, except to impress the patient. Shortage of time is not too much of a problem if data collection is spread over a number of visits.

In fact the main aim of both history and physical examination should be to record baselines against which to evaluate future events. These are much more likely than evidence of organ damage already present, or of some rare cause of secondary hypertension, whose detection is more an unlikely byproduct than a practical objective in its own right.

Patients should be asked routinely about sternal pain on exercise and 'indigestion' pains, about calf pain on walking or running, and about breathlessness. Paroxysmal nocturnal dyspnoea rarely has to be asked for — it presents readily enough because it is so frightening — but the other two often have to be actively elicited.

Patients should also be asked whether they have any symptoms which they themselves attribute to hypertension. This attribution is rarely correct, but it is important, particularly at this early stage, to know how patients themselves conceive of their 'disease', and to discuss this with them before the effects of antihypertensive drugs complicate matters.

There is little point in recording standing and lying pressures, unless there are positive reasons for suspecting autonomic neuropathy, as in diabetes and old age, or in patients complaining of faint spells.

Heart rhythm should be noted. A large heart is obvious in a few patients, and can be confirmed by chest X-ray. Unless there are symptoms of heart failure, or there is some other indication, routine chest radiography for all hypertensives is not helpful or necessary; nor is routine pyelography.

We do a routine ECG, chiefly in order to have a previous tracing available in the event of later chest pain. It is particularly useful always to know whether bundle branch block is old or recent; in the absence of this knowledge it may be impossible to interpret ECG evidence of infarction later on. We try to avoid overstatement of the prognostic value of ECGs to patients, who tend to have exaggerated faith in machinery of all kinds.

Lungs should be checked for crackles, and whether these clear on coughing. Peak expiratory flow rate should be recorded for all patients and matched against the predicted value for sex, age and height; all asthmatics, overt or latent, need to be identified before rather than after prescription of beta-blocking drugs.

The abdomen should be examined for palpable liver and kidneys, aortic aneurysm and reduced femoral pulses.

Carotid pulses should be felt and murmurs listened for posterior tibial and dorsalis pedis pulses should be noted, again mainly as baselines for future events.

Fundi should be examined once at an early stage, with pupils fully dilated with a mydriatic. Ninety-eight times out of 100 this is of value only as a baseline measurement, but it has to be done. A fleeting glance through an undilated pupil is a futile gesture.

LABORATORY TESTS

Urine should be tested for glucose and protein, and one dip-culture should be set up to screen for renal tract infection. In obese older patients with body mass index >30 or a family history of diabetes, we take blood for glycosylated haemoglobin (HbA1C) as a further screening test for diabetes.

We also ask for routine baseline measurements of blood electrolytes, urea, creatinine, urate, and gamma glutamyl transferase (gamma GT), and a full blood count for mean corpuscular volume (as another indicator of alcohol problems) and packed cell volume, an important risk factor for stroke.

ARE THERE OTHER COMPLICATING MEDICAL PROBLEMS?

Most of our patients over the age of 50 have some other major medical problem which complicates management of high blood pressure. For example, in 1983, 12 out of 25 adult diabetics also needed antihypertensive medication; about 30% of our hypertensives were obese with a body mass index >30, 12% of all men in the practice had a known alcohol problem, and 22% had a peak expiratory flow rate <300 l/min. This is one of the most important reasons why nearly all hypertensives should be managed by primary care generalists rather than either hospital specialists or (more realistically) junior hospital staff in training.

IS THERE A COMMON CAUSE OF SECONDARY HYPERTENSION?

Undergraduate teaching tends to leave the impression that the known causes of hypertension are rare, and since essential hypertension is by definition of unknown cause, there is no point in searching for common causes. Patients always wonder why their blood pressure is raised, and some effort to answer this question is worthwhile, apart from the most obvious of all, an evaluation of family history.

The contraceptive pill is one fairly common cause of secondary hypertension, which may be severe. It should be excluded in every hypertensive woman of reproductive age. She may be getting the pill from another source, such as the Family Planning Association. Pressure falls within a month or two of withdrawal. Other iatrogenic causes are carbenoxolone and large doses of sympathomimetic amines.

Although obesity generally makes only a small causal contribution to hypertension, and weight reduction has a correspondingly small effect in controlling it, this is not necessarily true of the individual case. Careful sequential measurements of blood pressure and weight may suggest that this is an important cause, and the feedback to the patient (in terms of reduced pressure) may be an important incentive to maintain weight control.

Alcohol is a common, important and reversible cause of hypertension which should be considered in every case, by taking a full alcohol history and checking mean corpuscular volume (MCV) and gamma GT. A full alcohol history means asking how much beer, wine or spirits is habitually taken on each day of a typical week.

Anxiety and depression

Depression (but not other psychiatric disorders) seems to be a frequent cause of hypertension. Blood pressure falls when affect improves. Unless pressure is sustained over a threshold of about 200/120 mmHg, or there is evidence of organ damage, antihypertensive drugs should not be used until depression resolves or is controlled. All antihypertensive drugs cause depression in some people, and this is rarely a risk worth taking.

Whether or not chronic anxiety causes sustained hypertension, acute anxiety and overwhelming personal problems certainly can raise pressure sufficiently to cause alarm to GPs, which may then be transmitted back to the patient, setting up a vicious circle which may receive a final twist by the hasty inception of antihypertensive drug treatment. Asking patients in a general way whether they have any worries is hardly ever effective. Patients worried out of their minds by a sick marriage, a child in trouble or bills that cannot be met, will not complicate their troubles by discussing them with you, unless they believe you can help. They are more likely to try to keep you out by denying any problems whatever, just as most of us answer the question 'How are you?' by 'Fine, thanks', however bad we feel. The approach must be more circumspect, with an eye for the patient who seems ill at ease or on the brink of tears. Often the best question is to ask them why they think their blood pressure might be raised. Material of this kind often comes out when the spouse is seen, as he or she should be at some point in the induction phase. As with depression, patients with acute anxieties rarely benefit from immediate treatment, and it is often best to agree to follow them up without treatment until they are coping better with their other problems, and then start medication.

Patients who, from evidence of previous contacts, are likely to complain of minor non-specific side-effects such as headache, tiredness or loss of libido may benefit from a couple of weeks on placebo before active medication begins, followed by open discussion of the results. Our experience is that patients afterwards accept this as a reasonable way of separating the effects of apprehension from drug-induced side-effects.

IS THERE A RARE CAUSE OF SECONDARY HYPERTENSION?

Some of the rarities are covered by your initial routine baseline measurements. Three-quarters of all cases of primary aldosteronism should turn up on an unexpectedly low serum potassium, though about a quarter have serum potassium within the normal range. If diagnosis is a guide to action rather than a puzzle for professional entertainment, the other quarter rarely matter, since impairment is caused either by hypokalaemia (which they have not got) or the hypertension itself, which can nearly always be readily controlled with antihypertensive medication (Swales 1983).

Coarctation of the aorta mostly presents in the first year of life, but those who survive this long rarely have symptoms thereafter until they get a stroke, go into heart failure, get subacute bacterial endocarditis, or rupture their aortae. They should turn up on routine search for foot and ankle pulses.

Polycystic kidneys should turn up on the family history, and most renal hypertension on a history of renal disease plus the results of your baseline measurements of blood urea, creatinine, and urate, and your search for proteinuria and bacteriuria. Chronic nephritis should be sought if you find chronic microhaematuria, which is present in about 10% of treated hypertensives in general practice (Ryan 1981), though few of these actually have a nephropathy. Routine pyelography in the absence of a history or renal disease is not justified. Of 952 routine pyelograms performed at the Glasgow MRC hypertension unit, 18% showed renal tract abnormalities but these influenced management in less than 1% (Atkinson & Kellett 1974).

Renal artery stenosis is a rare cause of hypertension. It is reversible by surgery in about 50% of cases; the rest still have to be controlled medically, so missing them is not the end of the world. Renal artery stenosis rarely causes symptoms unless it presents with the malignant phase, a renal infarct, or the hyponatraemic hypertensive syndrome, with thirst, polyuria, no glycosuria, and salt-craving. About half of all cases have an abdominal systolic murmur over the renal arteries, but the vast majority of such bruits are caused by atheroma rather than primary stenosis, and are a result rather than a cause of hypertension. So even this classical sign is fairly useless, and there is really no satisfactory screening test for this disorder. The Glasgow MRC Hypertension Research Unit (Mackay et al 1983) suggests two groups commonly seen by the GP in whom investigation could be reasonably cost-effective:

1. Patients who are young and have moderate or severe hypertension. They define 'young' as under 45. To this I would add: 'with a negative family history of hypertension and no alcohol problem'. This narrows the field very considerably, as hypertension in young men is fairly common, but nearly all cases have one or usually both parents with hypertension, or are heavy drinkers.
2. Compliant patients with treated hypertension whose blood pressure control rapidly and unexpectedly deteriorates.

Phaeochromocytoma is said to have a prevalence between 0.1 and 1% in the general population (Ball 1983). About 10% are familial and 5% are associated with neurofibromatosis; these get diagnosed sooner, otherwise most are diagnosed over the age of 40. The tumour releases a variable mixture of adrenaline (epinephrine) and noradrenaline (norepinephrine), sometimes continuously, sometimes intermittently. Classically there is unstable hypertension with paroxysmal symptoms of anxiety, sweating, tachycardia, palpitations, nausea, flushing, vomiting, and tremor. Hypertension is frequently sustained and stable, or if adrenaline release predominates, may not be present at all. The diagnosis may be suspected when high pressure is first recorded, or when response to treatment is erratic and incomprehensible.

Diagnosis is usually by measurement of degradation products of adrenaline and noradrenaline in 24-h samples of urine. If amine release is intermittent, so are the urinary concentrations of their metabolites, so urine collection should begin when the patient first feels characteristic symptoms. The most widely available test is for vanil mandelic acid (VMA), though this seems to be less sensitive and specific than free catecholamines and normetanephrine. Bananas, coffee, tea, chocolate, vanilla, phenolic drugs like aspirin, and citrus fruits should all be excluded from the diet from the time that the urine collection begins, as all can give false high values for VMA. Several tests may be necessary before you pick up the tumour, and if you really suspect it, persistence pays. Routine screening is not effective, and nearly all suspected cases turn out to be anxious people with panic attacks.

Cushing's syndrome (glucocorticoid excess) is equally rare, and causes hypertension in about three-quarters of all cases (Kaplan 1983). Its appearance is familiar because of the hypercortical facies of steroid treatment. The diagnosis is confirmed by the dexamethasone suppression test — measurement of plasma cortisol the day following a bedtime dose of 1 mg dexamethasone.

REFERRAL

No doubt GPs still exist who refer all cases of hypertension to a district hospital for assessment, treatment and follow-up, but they will not be reading this book. Who needs referral, and what should be done at the other end?

The question is serious. Relatively few hospital specialists are really interested in hypertension, and except in these innovating centres, district hospital physicians, even cardiologists, rarely have much more to give than GPs, apart from more time, a bigger team, and perhaps more direct access to the laboratory and X-ray department. Many have to cope with too many uncomplicated hypertensives to be able to give special attention to the truly difficult cases, whose greatest need is usually a larger number of readings and better assessment of compliance to find out what is really going on. The GP is probably better placed than most specialists to carry out these simple enquiries.

Three groups rally need referral:

1. Young hypertensives, say under the age of 35, if they have a negative family history;
2. People whose blood pressure cannot be controlled after 3 months or more with a double or treble drug combination most of whom are either not taking their tablets or are drinking too much alcohol, but including a few with secondary hypertension;
3. People with major organ damage, for example heart failure or renal failure, needing specialised advice in its own right.

In some of these cases referral to a regional centre may be necessary for ambulatory intra-arterial blood pressure monitoring.

WHAT RESOURCES AND LIMITATIONS DOES THE PATIENT HAVE?

At some point close to the inception of treatment, patient and spouse should be seen together to discuss a long-term plan for management. This should include not only antihypertensive medication, with discussion of possible side-effects, but also plans for changes in diet and perhaps smoking and drinking. Social and occupational difficulties should be discussed, and an informal contract for treatment agreed upon, which takes into account both the resources available to the patient, and the limitations he or she perceives.

Plans must be realistic. Doctors are poor judges of what patients can or cannot do; they are unable to predict who will succeed and who will fail in adhering to a treatment plan, and contrary to medical folklore, no sociodemographic variables show any consistent association with compliance (Haynes 1977). We do know, however, that GPs can do rather better than hospitals in securing compliance (Drury et al 1976), and that patients do best if they have a share in devising treatment plans themselves.

SUGGESTED SEQUENCE FOR EARLY DATA COLLECTION

First (identification) visit

Arrange for repeat blood pressure measurements on at least two more separate days, then if mean pressure warrants it, arrange second visit.

Second visit

Family history of stroke, coronary disease, diabetes, and causes of death in parents and siblings.

Current symptoms, especially those attributed by the patient to hypertension.

Current medication, especially oral contraception and antidepressants.

Baseline ECG, peak expiratory flow rate (PEFR), ankle and foot pulses, funduscopy, urine for glucose and protein, examination of heart and lungs, height, weight, blood for full blood count (FBC), biochemical screen including urea, creatinine, urate, total cholesterol and gamma GT, glycosylated haemoglobin (HbAlc) if BMI = >35 or there is a family history of diabetes.

Third visit

Review results of baseline measurements. If total cholesterol is

6.5 mmol/dl or over, arrange for fasting lipid profile. If MCV = >95 or there is high triglyceride or gamma GT, search again for high alcohol intake.

Take a diet history concentrating on fat and alcohol.

Record current exercise at home and at work, past and potential future interests in exercise.

Are there any major problems at home or at work? Ask specifically about sex function.

Fourth visit

Arrange for the spouse to accompany the patient.

Discuss investigation results, agree a plan for control of other coronary and stroke risk factors.

Take a decision to:

> review blood pressure annually, or
>
> teach patient or spouse to do home recordings and return in 2 weeks with 28 readings, or
>
> initiate antihypertensive medication and return to follow-up clinic in 4 weeks.

REFERENCES

Atkinson A B, Kellett R J 1974 Value of intravenous urography in investigating hypertension. Journal of the Royal College of Physicians of London 8:175

Ball S G 1983 Phaeochromocytoma. In: Robertson J I S (ed) Handbook of Hypertension vol 2. Clinical aspects of secondary hypertension. Elsevier Science Publishers, Oxford, p 238

Drury V W M, Wade O L, Woolf E 1976 Following advice in general practice. Journal of the Royal College of General Practitioners 26:712

Haynes R B A critical review of the determinants of patient compliance with therapeutic regimens. In: Sackett D L, Haynes R B (eds) Compliance with therapeutic regimens. Johns Hopkins University Press, Baltimore, p 26

Kaplan N M 1983 Cushing's syndrome and hypertension. In: Robertson J I S (ed) Handbook of Hypertension vol 2. Clinical aspects of secondary hypertension. Elsevier Science Publishers, Oxford, p 208

Mackay A, Brown J J, Lever A F et al 1983 Unilateral renal disease in hypertension. In: Robertson J I S (ed) Handbook of hypertension vol 2. Clinical aspects of secondary hypertension. Elsevier Science Publishers, Oxford, p 33

Parkin D M, Kellett R J, Maclean D W et al 1979 The management of hypertension: a study of records in general practice. Journal of the Royal College of General Practitioners 22:590

Ryan W A 1981 Microscopic haematuria in hypertension. Lancet ii:994

Swales J D 1983 Primary aldosteronism: how hard should we look? British Medical Journal 287:702

13

Organisation of follow-up

Clinical medicine in the sense of traditional puzzle-solving is important and great fun, but it has hardly anything to do with successful control of hypertension and its associated risk factors in large numbers of people. Starting with a complete population screen in 1968–1970, and using a treatment threshold of diastolic 105 mmHg revised to 100 mmHg in 1980 and back to 105 mmHg in 1985 (plus patients with organ damage and diabetes), applied to a population of 1700–2000, in Glyncorrwg we normally manage about 130 hypertensives. These patients are seen once every 3 months if they are well controlled, more often if not, so we are talking about the organisation of at least 600 visits a year.

CLINIC OR JUMBLE?

Many GPs are opposed in principle to special clinics in general practice, and I have much sympathy with their view. They believe that any and all clinics sooner or later degenerate into impersonal, over-structured conveyor belts, in which a fixed series of delegated standard procedures are performed by a nurse, while the doctor signs forms. I have known clinics like this, and refused to segregate care of hypertensives in my own practice as long as possible because of the same fears.

About 3 years after our screening was completed we did our first team audit on care of hypertensives. The results were appalling. Many patients were rediscovered who had either lapsed from treatment altogether, or were collecting repeat prescriptions without any medical supervision. We set up first a monthly and later a fortnightly clinic, with a check on defaulters at the end of each session and a full audit once a year. Since then our compliance and control figures have been as good as or better than any figures reported from teaching hospitals, although unlike theirs, our results are based on a whole population on an intention-to-treat basis. If those who oppose clinics in general practice can achieve 80% control (blood pressure <160/90 mmHg) and 80% compliance (treated patients seen within a 4-month span and all untreated patients at least once a year), good luck to them; but we couldn't do it, and I doubt if many of my colleagues can.

The position is analogous to antenatal care, which until the 1950s was often scattered through the jumble of patient demand, and presented the same problems of ensuring that a minimum standard of care be achieved and regular contact maintained. Antenatal clinics, particularly the fully industrialised ones in hospitals, can be insensitive and inhuman, but the answer to that is not to abolish them, but to keep them small, flexible, personal, and in the community. The best GP antenatal clinics are a good and familiar model for what is needed in GP hypertension clinics.

It is impossible even to try to confine all hypertension-related consultations to the clinic, or to confine the clinic consultations to hypertension and its related risks. If hypertensive patients for some reason consult a week or so before their clinic day, it is petty to insist they they come again for a blood pressure check; and if, during a hypertension clinic, patients have other problems they want to discuss, reasonable flexibility should be shown in accepting them. If you don't do this, compliance will fall. We find that about 25% of our hypertension consultations, including all the induction phase, occur outside our clinic structure.

How often?

We operate on a 3-monthly cycle, not only for hypertension follow-up, but also for oral contraception monitoring and follow-up of most chronic disease and long-term certification. We find this simple to remember for both staff and patients and it fits in with reasonable quantities for repeat medication. Roughly 20% of patients booked in to a clinic don't come; about half of them because they have already been seen in a jumble session, the other half because they have forgotten, work impossible hours, or are persistent defaulters. This means that with a 3-month cycle, about 10% of the patients are actually seen on a 4-month or even 5-month cycle.

Some practices operate a 6-month cycle, and this will reduce workload. Even on a 3-month cycle, a high proportion of cases, at least 20%, have pressures above target level, and I do not believe we could extend our cycle without impairing quality of care.

How many patients?

We book about 20 patients for each follow-up session, of whom 15 to 18 turn up. About two-thirds of these are dealt with entirely by the nurse, and of the other third who want to see the doctor, about half have hypertension-related problems (usually poor control), and the rest have some other problem. The hypertension clinic is run concurrently with an ordinary jumble session, so that from the doctor's point of view, the feared monotomy of special clinics cannot arise.

Which staff?

The bare essentials are a nurse and a doctor. Undoubtedly, a nurse who follows a logical plan for continuing care is safer and better than a doctor who doesn't, and there are cases where individual nurses have more of the qualities needed for innovation than any doctor available in the group. However, these are exceptional, and there are as many job-and-finish nurses as there are doctors; in general, both doctors and nurses are needed for an effective clinic.

It is important to remember that divisions of labour within the team should change over time, as members of staff gain confidence and experience, and develop new skills and interests. All members of the team should be encouraged both to read and to contribute to the professional literature at an appropriate level, and none should continue in post longer than 2 years without going away for some kind of further training, even if it's just a one-day conference.

For educational work, particularly on associated risk factors, more people are needed, preferably less professionalised. The point is fully discussed in Chapter 11.

SIX CONDITIONS FOR COMPLIANCE

Studies in the USA have shown that up to 50% of people who identified as hypertensives fail even to enter the treatment and follow-up pipeline, another 50% drop out of care within the first year, and over 30% of those who remain fail to take enough medication to control pressure (Sackett & Snow 1979).

To maximise compliance, there are six preconditions ('six Cs'): Credulity, Continuity, Concern, Comprehension, Contract and eConomy.

Credulity

Doctors who think they can predict who will not be 'a good patient' are wrong; studies have shown that apart from extremes of age, no sociodemographic variables are consistently associated with either compliance or non-compliance (Menard et al 1900; Haynes 1977), and doctors are very poor predictors of patient behaviour (Mushlin & Appel 1977). So the first condition for maximal compliance is an open mind; all patients who really need antihypertensive treatment, from archbishops to alcoholics, should be offered it.

Continuity and concern

Finnerty et al (1973) studied drop-outs from a US inner city outpatient clinic. He reduced the annual drop-out rate from 42% to less than 4% in 2 years and 85% of these subjects now have blood pressures at or below target, so his conclusions are worth listening to.

> We rapidly learned that patients dropped out not because they were uneducated or did not care about their health, and not because they could not afford the medication. Rather, they abandoned the clinic because they were treated like cattle, herded from one room to another, left waiting for hours, then examined by a different doctor on each visit, leaving no opportunity to develop any kind of relationship. . . The average waiting time for the doctor was 2.5 hours, and the average waiting time for drugs at the pharmacy was another 1.8 hours. . . In contrast. . . the average time actually spent with the physician was only 7.5 minutes.

Finnerty's solution was to reorganise the clinic by developing an effective appointments system (average time spent by patients in the clinic fell from 4 h to 20 min), and by ensuring continuity of staff–patient relationships. This turned out to be more important than staff qualification.

> Most important was the assignment of every patient to his or her own paramedic whom he would see on every visit. The paramedics frequently came from the same neighbourhood as the patient. . . chosen not so much because of [their] prior experience or education but because of [their] friendly and sympathetic personality and ability to identify with the patients.

Perfunctory care has perfunctory results. If we want patients to show effective concern for their health, we must show effective concern ourselves, by ensuring both continuity of care and a flow rate that allows time to listen and to explain.

Comprehension

Antihypertensive drugs vary in many ways, but they have one feature in common; none of them work when dropped into the toilet. Whether people take their medication, and whether they attend for follow-up, depends above all on their own system of beliefs about health and disease in general, and high blood pressure in particular.

Studies of hypertensives attending clinics in Baltimore showed that 92% were unaware that even very high blood pressure rarely caused symptoms, 81% were unaware of any possible side-effects from their medication (Williamson et al 1975), and 97% thought that the word 'hypertension' meant 'worry, tension, or nerves' (Green et al 1975). Of 42 patients seen in a Detroit hospital with a hypertensive emergency, 39% had been on antihypertensive treatment which they had stopped because they felt well (Caldwell et al 1970). Since people in Britain are generally less well informed about cardiovascular risks than people in the USA, the consequences of these myths probably apply here with even greater force.

Patients fear the diagnosis of hypertension, but except in the tiny minority in whom immediate fear is justified, fear is a bad motive for compliance. Patients quickly discover that whatever fortuitous symptoms first brought them to the doctor have disappeared, and from then on they feel better without medication and without supervision. From this they soon conclude that if they feel better untreated, they are better untreated. 'Hypertension' must be replaced by 'high blood pressure', with an explanation of exactly what that does and does not mean. Patients have to learn the falsity of disease labelling and dogmatic certainties, and the value of risk reduction and inquisitive doubt, preferably by considering their own personal data ranked in a population distribution.

Contract

The informed patient begins to be in a position to negotiate an unwritten but nevertheless real contract. The primary care team has a few rules which patients must observe if they want to receive care, but we must respect the right of patients to a continuing explanation of what we are doing, why we are doing it, what the consequences of doing it may be, and to choose alternatives where they exist. For example, we do not have the right to start a man on thiazide diuretics without explaining that this may cause erectile failure, that if this occurs it will stop when the drug is withdrawn, and that plenty of alternative drugs exist. It is not possible or desirable to make patients responsible for decisions which they rightly consider to be our responsibility, but a start must be made in involving patients in more of these decisions if we want them to take a more active role in their own treatment.

This is particularly important for the minority of patients who reject treatment, either from the start, or by systematic non-compliance. It must be made clear to them that a decision not to accept treatment is not a decision to reject all supervision. Most will accept at least an annual check, with renewed negotiation if pressure rises substantially.

Economy

Simplicity of drugs and dosage is essential for high compliance. There are no major groups of antihypertensive drugs that require more than twice-daily dosage, and most cases can now be controlled with once-daily dosage, often with two drugs in fixed combination. It is worth remembering that the highly successful Veterans Administration trials relied on one pill a day of combined thiazide and reserpine. GPs are more aware than hospital doctors of the problems arising when patients on treble antihypertensive medication also have to take two, three, or even more other drugs concurrently to control other problems, such as diabetes or airways obstruction.

THREE COMPONENTS OF FOLLOW-UP

Hypertension and its management last for the rest of the patient's life. From the time that a single high pressure reading is obtained, to the time when organ failure or intercurrent disease brings super-vision to an end, follow-up has three components: a complex induction phase of baseline investigation, patient education, and initial trial of treatment; a simple continuing phase of monitoring on a 3-monthly or other regular cycle, usually with a healthy patient; and an organ-damage phase in which treatment becomes complex again, new variables must be monitored, and patients begin to be sick.

The induction phase

There is so much to do in the induction phase that separation from long-term follow-up is essential. If your appointment system is run fairly tightly, you are not likely to have more than 10 minutes even for induction consultations, so these meetings must be spread out over at least three visits, often five or six, ending at the point where a treatment plan has been formulated and begun, and thereafter need only be modified to achieve targets for pressure and other risk factors.

The main tasks of the induction phase have been discussed earlier, and here it may be more useful to set them out in note form, starting from the first high pressure recorded, and ending with the start of a management plan:

Verification. Repeat blood pressure at least three times on separate visits to practice nurse. Even then it may be difficult to decide whether medication is justified. Consider teaching the patient or a relative to make home measurements with an electronic sphygmomanometer and arrange for twice-daily readings for 2 weeks before next visit.

History. First, significant to you: shortness of breath, chest pain, leg pain, renal tract symptoms now or in the past, gout, depressive symptoms including loss of libido, other current or previous illnesses, and family history. Then, chiefly for their significance to the patient: headache, palpitation, and what do you think might be the cause of your high blood pressure?

Management setting. The family, work, and other social environment within which management plans will be constrained. All, or nearly all the information required should already be there in a good record; but is it? The spouse will be your best source of data of this kind.

Examination.   Fundi (dilated)
Eyes for corneal arcus
Carotid and ankle pulses
Heart sounds and apex
Lungs for crackles and wheezes
Peak flow rate
Fingers for tobacco

Hands, face and belly for alcohol
Weight and height
ECG

Side-room tests.
  Urine dipstick for glucose, protein etc.
  Urine dip-culture for bacteriuria

Blood tests. All tests except HDL cholesterol can be done on casual samples of blood. HDL cholesterol may require blood after a 12 h fast (though experts differ about this). If you can be really sure the patient will do it, all the blood samples can then be taken in one go (using Vacutainers) together with the fasting sample. If you decide that a bird in the hand is worth two in the bush, put off the fasting sample till later. Altogether you will want:

Urea and creatinine
Urate
Gamma GT
Potassium

All the above should be obtainable together on one 10 ml centri-fuged clotted sample through an auto-analyser.

Blood for total cholesterol may need to be taken separately.
  Haemoglobin, packed cell volume, mean cell volume.
  HbAlc (in sequestrene container) if you have any
  reason to suspect diabetes.
  Casual blood alcohol (in fluoride container) with
  time of collection noted, if you have any reason
  to suspect an alcohol problem.
  Fasting lipid profile (10 ml clotted).

Education. This falls into four parts:
  The nature of hypertension as an
  asymptomatic risk factor;
  The patient's personal risk profile for
  arterial disease;
  The patient's attitudes, resources and
  constraints within which a management
  plan must be formulated;
  The management plan. This must include
  explanation of probable and possible
  side-effects of drugs, duration of
  management (usually for life), and
  understanding of an informal contract.

A lot to do. How these tasks should be divided, over time and between staff, needs to be agreed within the team. Though in general patients remember more if consultation times are fairly short, it is a great advantage if every patient has at least one early opportunity for a long session of about 20 minutes, for an extended discussion. Back-up with written material is helpful, and as this must not conflict with team policy, it is usually best to produce this locally, perhaps by modifying centrally published material, for example that offered in Appendices I, XI and XII of this book. Every practice needs access to a duplicator; schools are usually helpful about this.

The continuing phase

Once a management plan has begun, follow-up visits have a smaller and more predictable content, easily contained within a 5-minute appointment time for the nurse, plus another 5–10 minutes with the doctor if targets are not reached or the patient wants to discuss other problems. We aim at an eventual 3-month cycle, but patients are seen weekly for dosage changes until target pressure is attained, and monthly if, having achieved target control, this is subsequently lost.

Our default target pressure is <160/90 mmHg. In a few patients this cannot be attained without intolerable side-effects, and you may have to settle for something higher, and try again later. The patient needs to know what the target is.

Patients see the nurse for measurement of blood pressure, weight, a check on smoking, and a positive search for medication side-effects. Control of smoking, unless it is attained quickly during the induction phase, fits awkwardly into schematic management. Similar ambiguities surround weight and blood cholesterol control. Techniques for control of weight, cholesterol and smoking within a follow-up programme are discussed in Chapter 14. Other variables, for example gamma GT, MCV or PEFR may be added to the standard package for individual patients for whom there are special indications.

Patients should always be asked to bring all their current medication with them. We find that fews patients learn the names of their drugs, despite encouragement to do so, and the safest way to discuss individual drugs is to have them there on the table. Medication for other conditions is easily forgotten unless this is done. Formal tablet counts are not an effective way of monitoring compliance because patients who are systematically non-compliant soon get wise to them, but a rough comparison of actual numbers in the bottle against those expected, without a formal count, can be a good indicator.

Periodic review

Several variables need monitoring occasionally, but less often than every 3 months. If patients seem well controlled and feel well, we aim to check urine for glucose and protein, and blood urea, creatinine, urate and potassium once every 5 years.

Drop-out review

At the end of each clinic session, doctor and nurse spend 5 minutes going through the non-attenders, discussing reasons for default and what should be done about it. This is the main opportunity for continuing education and modification of the control programme in the light of experience. Once every 3 months, the nurse should go through the whole card-box of hypertensives, whether treated or observed, together with their GP records; errors will always be found, and they need chasing up before rot sets in.

The organ-damaged phase

Sooner or later most treated hypertensives will develop evidence of organ damage, most commonly angina and claudication, often diabetes and occasionally early renal failure which will initially be asymptomatic. Management of these conditions is discussed fully in Chapter 18. Monitoring of the management of these complications can either be added on to the standard tasks of the clinic, or the complications can be dealt with separately at ordinary jumble sessions while continuing to monitor blood pressure at the clinic. It is usually a mistake to remove anyone from the clinic completely, because some kind of follow-up is always needed, and jumble sessions are not organised to detect default.

ENTRIES, EXITS AND INTERRUPTIONS

Once a system is running, it must include provision for treated hypertensives moving in from other practices, moving out, or temporarily removed. In each case it is important that management should not lapse.

Once high blood pressure is well controlled, there is usually no clinical evidence that it ever existed. Antihypertensive treatment on inadequate criteria is so common that treatment may easily be allowed to lapse by a critical GP when a patient moves, with too short a follow-up period to detect a dangerous rise in pressure. This may take as long as 6 months to reappear after treatment is lapsed, and the average delay in receiving a patient's previous medical record from the Family Practitioner Committee, containing the original evidence for treatment, is 3 months. Patients transferring in should usually be placed in your own clinic and followed up for about 6 months before considering any trial of no medication. If this is done, monitoring every 3 months is essential for the first year, and annually thereafter.

Patients leaving the practice should be given a letter for the new GP including the original criteria for treatment as well as details of current medication.

Admission to hospital all too frequently interrupts or revises and complicates treatment and may cause it to lapse altogether. Most anaesthetists now aim to continue blood pressure control during the operative period; to withdraw antihypertensive drugs preoperatively from a moderate or severe hypertensive is as rational as withdrawal of insulin from a diabetic (Edwards 1979). Even so, medication is often changed, without explanation or return to original medication on discharge, leading to unnecessary and occasionally dangerous confusion. Where medication is stopped, it is often not re-started before leaving hospital, and patients may not understand that a surgical house officer usually knows and perhaps cares less about management of hypertension than their own family doctor. Difficulties also arise with medical departments, which may switch medication to whatever drugs their unit favours, without regard to your own practice policy, thus thoroughly confusing the patient. It is particularly important to make sure that previous evidence of airways obstruction is known, so that beta-blockers will not be used if they are contraindicated. Patients should take only 1 or 2 days' medication with them to hospital when they are admitted. If they bring in whole bottles these will only be thrown away; despite the present poverty of the Health Service, medication removed on admission is never (in my experience) returned to patients when they leave.

ANNUAL AUDIT

We aim to review all our cases once a year, on the following variables:

What proportion of clinic patients is at or below target pressure (<160/90 mmHg)?

How does the group mean pre-medication pressure (mean of the last three readings before medication began) compare with the current group mean pressure (mean of the last three available readings)?

What proportion had body mass index <30 when medication began, and what proportion does now?

What proportion smoked when medication began, and what proportion does now?

What proportion of medicated cases has been seen and reviewed within the last 4 months?

What proportion of observed cases has been seen and reviewed within the past year?

I have called this 'annual' review, but in fact we have done it erratically, about once every 3 years, because without computerisation the procedure is so laborious. Once data are computerised you can do this any time.

THE CLINIC AS A SOCIAL GROUP

One of the most precious advantages of concentrating cases in a clinic is that the patients get to know one another as people with a shared problem. They will begin to educate one another, as already happens with diabetics; studies a generation ago showed clearly that diabetics get most of their knowledge from other diabetics rather than directly from doctors or nurses. It also means that the patients can from time to time be convened as a group, to discuss organisation of care or new developments in management of hypertension and associated risk factors.

REFERENCES

Caldwell J R, Cobb S, Dowling M D et al 1970 The dropout problem in antihypertensive treatment: a pilot study of social and emotional factors influencing a patient's ability to follow antihypertensive treatment. Journal of Chronic Diseases 22:579

Edwards W T 1979 Preanaesthetic management of the hypertensive patient. New England Journal of Medicine 301:158

Finnerty F A, Mattie E C, Finnerty F A 1973 Hypertension in the inner city. I. Analysis of drop-outs. Circulation 47:73

Green L W, Levine D M, Deeds S 1975 Clinical trials of health education for hypertensive outpatients: design and baseline data. Preventive Medicine 4:417

Haynes R B 1977 A critical review of the determinants of patient compliance with therapeutic regimens. In: Sackett D L, Haynes R B (eds) Compliance with therapeutic regimens, Johns Hopkins University Press, Baltimore, p 26

Menard J, Degoulet P, Hong A V et al 1983 Compliance in hypertension care. In: Gross F, Strasser T (eds) Mild hypertension: recent advances. Raven Press, New York.

Mushlin A I, Appel F A 1977 Diagnosing patient non-compliance. Archives of Internal Medicine 137:318

Sackett D L, Snow J S 1979 The magnitude of compliance and non-compliance. In: Haynes R B, Taylor D W, Sackett D L (eds) Compliance in health care. Johns Hopkins University Press, Baltimore, p 11

Williamson J W, Aaronovitch S, Simonson L et al 1975 Health accounting: an outcome-based system of quality assurance: illustrative application to hypertension. Bulletin of the New York Academy of Medicine 51:727

14

Management without drugs: sodium restriction, weight control, glucose intolerance and alcohol

Traditionally, management by behavioural change has been seen as an alternative or an adjunct to antihypertensive medication for controlling blood pressure alone, and efficacy has been judged only in terms of pressure reduction. There is a case for dietary change and relaxation techniques in controlling mild or moderate high blood pressure as a single risk (Andrews et al 1982), but the argument is much stronger and more interesting if we consider control of all major risk factors, as the MRC trial logically compels us to do.

It has also been generally assumed that personalised education for behavioural change in high risk groups is a separate world entirely from behavioural change in the community as a whole. In the uniquely British debate over the justifications for and feasibility of any planned action on a population scale to prevent coronary disease (Oliver 1983; Hart 1985), protagonists on both sides protest that they do not wish to pitch individual care against collective change as alternative and opposed strategies. In practice, however, this is precisely what most of them do. There are several reasons for this, the most important of which is British economic decline, with consequent abdication from social responsibilities which were once taken for granted. While still assuming its own natural right to the best of everything, including anticipatory and preventive medical care, noblesse no longer obliges. Personalised preventive care is now being energetically and uncritically pursued for a small wealthy minority, but all that is done for the mass of the people is to set up committees to agonise over whether prevention is either feasible or effective.

British social class differences in mortality are now greater than they have ever been since figures became available early this century. In Sweden these differences have now disappeared, proving that with a different set of social priorities the job can be done. Britain now has the highest age-specific coronary death rates and all-causes death rates in western Europe, the lowest proportion of gross national product devoted to health and medical care, and the highest per capita spending on preparation for war. Because of the size of the populations involved, even a high risk strategy, confined say to the top five centiles of combined risk, is a mass strategy if fully applied. It would therefore demand new resources which cannot be filched from other parts of an already impoverished service. To win against competing social pressures, its advocates require more than gentlemanly expertise; they must learn either to think in terms of new social alliances, or accept defeat.

Primary care is the site at which it is possible to unite control of high blood pressure with control of other risks, unite high risk with mass strategies, and unite personalised advice with group and community action. It is also perhaps the most feasible growing point for participative democracy. Providing they have the courage and imagination to move forward rather than backward, family doctors could help to create a uniquely exciting and effective future in precisely this area.

In this chapter we will consider each of the main non-pharmacological measures that have been used both to lower blood pressure and to reduce other risk factors.

DIETARY SODIUM

Evidence that high dietary sodium is a main cause of hypertension has already been discussed in Chapter 3. Experimental evidence that this is so remains poor, but is also difficult to obtain. Indeed if, as some suggest, sodium overload must operate throughout the first 5 or 10 years of life to cause high blood pressure, proof by controlled experiment may be impossible. Circumstantial evidence in favour of sodium overload as a cause of hypertension remains strong despite its generally poor quality, but the argument should become much clearer when the Intersalt studies are completed.

In this chapter, however, we are concerned not with causation, but with the effect of low-sodium diet on raised blood pressure and other cardiovascular risk factors.

How high or low are we talking about?

Sodium and potassium are discussed in this book in terms of SI units (millimoles). Conversion from grams is as follows:

1 g NaCl = 17.1 mmol Na
1 g Na   = 43.5 mmol Na
1 g KCl = 13.4 mmol K
1 g K   = 25.6 mmol K

Surveys of British food habits suggest an average adult intake of about 200 mmol/day sodium (Bull & Buss 1980), though research studies on small populations have mostly shown lower intakes around 150 mmol/day for men and 130 mmol/day for women. It is worth bearing in mind that big people eat more of everything than little people, and therefore eat more sodium; the average man is bigger than the average woman. This quantity is about 10 times the minimum physiological requirement, and three or four times the average for groups in Polynesia, rural Africa and South America which have no hypertension and no rise in blood pressure with age. On the other hand, it is about 50% less than the sodium load in northern Japan, 40% less than in Portugal, and 25% less than in Belgium, Australia and the USA.

Because sodium glutamate is added to many processed foods to improve flavour (bringing Chinese take-away meals to monstrous sodium loads of 200 mmol or more per portion), sodium nitrite is added as a preservative, and the entire food industry is competing for instant flavour-appeal, processed foods are now the main (and not always obvious) source of dietary sodium. De Swiet (1982) gives examples; one average-sized potato contains 0.2 mmol sodium compared with 21 mmol in one cupful of instant mashed potato; one portion of branded fried chicken contains 75 mmol, and one portion of branded hamburger and chips contains 97 mmol.

A sodium intake below the physiological minimum will control malignant hypertension, but above a threshold of 10 mmol daily the diet is ineffective (MRC 1950). Serious sodium restriction has always been difficult, and with the advent of thiazide diuretics which seemed to do the same job painlessly, English-speaking doctors quickly lost interest in dietary sodium restriction, though the idea persisted in continental Europe.

Though the ground was prepared by Dahl's persuasive arguments on causation based on his rats and between-society comparisons, the paper which first revived interest in sodium restriction as a treatment in Britain and the USA was from Morgan et al in Australia in 1978. He studied hospital outpatients with a before-trial mean daily intake of 195 mmol sodium. Experimental subjects were given a target of 100 mmol/day, and controls were given no dietary advice. Two years later the experimental subjects were found to have a group mean diastolic pressure 7 mmHg less than the controls, and this was generally accepted as evidence that moderate sodium restriction was an effective treatment. In fact the experimental subjects only achieved a group mean daily sodium intake of 157 mmol, the design was not blind, and controls had their blood pressures measured less often than the experimental subjects, an obvious potential source of difference in pressure. The news of this treatment, so powerful that it worked even if it was only 45% applied, made rapid headway through international medical opinion. In no time at all advice on sodium restriction became a necessary part of what every good physician claimed to be doing.

Does it work?

Two double-blind controlled trials have shown no effect on blood pressure in normotensives (Puska et al 1983) or borderline hypertensives (Watt et al 1983) when sodium restriction to 60–80 mmol/day was sustained for 4 weeks, and I am not aware of any similar studies conflicting with this. Results are no better with very young subjects; in a randomised crossover trial, Cooper et al (1984) found no effect from reduction of dietary sodium from 110 to 45 mmol/day for 24 days in 124 normotensive adolescents with a mean age of 16 years. One non-blind randomised trial of sodium restriction to 117 mmol/day showed no effect on blood pressure after 3 months in mild hypertensives (mean blood pressure 163/98 mmHg; Silman et al 1983).

However, measurable effects seem to appear in subjects with higher pressures — 'real' hypertensives. Studying hypertensives with a mean supine diastolic pressure of 98 mmHg after a 2-month run-in period, McGregor et al (1982) obtained a 7 mmHg fall in mean pressure after 4 weeks of sodium restriction to 86 mmol in a randomised double-blind trial.

Two conclusions are reasonable from the few adequately designed and performed trials so far available. The first is that sodium restriction to 50–80 mmol/day has no useful effect on normal or borderline high blood pressure over short periods of 4 weeks or so. We have no evidence either way on longer periods, but it is surely interesting that reduction of dietary fat (discussed below) does have a measurable effect within 4 weeks, so why not sodium?

The second is that moderate and severe hypertensives do show a fall in pressure with sodium restriction below 80 mmol/day, which seems to be directly proportional to the severity of their hypertension (Parfrey et al 1981). The pressure threshold for this effect seems to lie above any accepted threshold for treatment, and no study so far has shown a big enough reduction in pressure from sodium restriction alone to achieve target pressures <160/90 mmHg without medication. This means that the therapeutic role of sodium restriction is not as an alternative to medication for control of mild hypertension, but as an adjunct to medication for moderate and severe hypertension.

Is it feasible?

Once we have overcome the problems of mass screening and ascertainment, the main obstacles to effective control of high blood pressure in populations is low compliance and high drop-out. Compliance falls and drop-out increases as we make greater and more complex demands on patients to make radical changes in their behaviour. Some of these, such as stopping smoking and reducing dietary fat, are necessary, effective, and backed up by consistent evidence, though insistence on them certainly impairs compliance with the easy, pill-taking part of the package. In deciding whether to add sodium restriction to these other tasks, we need to know how big a burden it is.

I know of no studies expressly designed to answer this question, but many who have conducted sodium restriction studies have expressed opinions on how easy or difficult it was for their experimental subjects. At one extreme Beard et al (1982) reported little difficulty in getting patients to reduce sodium intake from 150 to 37 mmol/day for 12 weeks; drop-outs from his study were no more in the unrestricted controls than in the experimental subjects. His paper makes no comment on any difficulties in maintaining compliance, and even refers to an 'elevation of mood' in the salt-restricted subjects, who achieved sodium intakes within the range of hunter-gatherer populations among whom hypertension is unknown; 67% of them said they intended to carry on with the diet indefinitely. MacGregor, who has run several tightly designed and controlled studies of sodium restriction on hospital-referred hypertensives, has written (1983) that 'moderate sodium restriction (reducing sodium intake to 70 mmol a day) can be quite easily achieved'.

On the other hand, other researchers have admitted to serious difficulty in maintaining compliance with 'moderate' sodium restriction. In the North Karelia coronary heart disease prevention project (Nissinen et al 1982), normotensive and hypertensive random samples from the general population were studied intensively during a big whole-population campaign to reduce sodium load from an initial mean daily intake of 215 mmol for men and 171 mmol for women. Advice to reduce dietary sodium without specific advice on how to implement this resulted in no change at all after 1 year, but after specific advice on methods was given, a 20% reduction was achieved. Hypertensives were given a 1-month trial of complete exclusion of salt from their food, and they achieved a 30–50% reduction in sodium load, but after the trial month original sodium loads were quickly regained. After 3 years of mass education, more intensive and on a bigger scale than anywhere else in the world, a general reduction of 20–25% was achieved, but this still left mean intakes higher than the average level in Britain, and over twice the target levels of 'moderate restriction' studies.

Our experience of three sodium restriction studies in Glyncorrwg, involving middle-aged hypertensives and relatively young people with hypertensive parents (minimum age 12 years) was that compliance with our target (<60 mmol/day) was difficult, though it was based on simple and specific dietary advice, families were helped by free provision of specially prepared low-sodium foods, and were individually supported by the research team on a scale that would be impossible in ordinary practice. When we asked our subjects what they thought about their 8-week experience of sodium restriction to a mean 50 mmol/day, all but one subject said that they found it difficult and unpleasant, and were glad to return to normal eating. The only exception, who claimed restriction was easy, we knew (from our measurements of urine sodium) to have been totally non-compliant.

It is impossible to reconcile these two views of how easy or difficult it is for people to reduce dietary sodium to 'natural' levels of 30–80 mmol/day. Social selection is certainly important, and I find the negative studies of screened populations more convincing than positive studies of referred or volunteer patients. All our research team restricted their own sodium intake for a week before starting the trials, and all of us found it very difficult. All the researchers I know of who have reported negative results have done so reluctantly; when they designed their studies, they hoped and believed that sodium restriction would be so effective for primary prevention. So I do not believe they are biased in their conclusion that sodium restriction below 80 mmol/day presents real difficulties to most patients. If it is so easy to restrict dietary sodium, why are there still so few published trials of high quality?

Can it be harmful?

Perfunctory advice to reduce salt, without verification or follow-up, is both harmless and ineffective. Serious advice, with specific reccomendations, written back-up, follow-up and verification by measurements of 24 h urine sodium, could be harmful if it confuses patients about the relative priority they should give to competing claims for difficult changes in behaviour. Even taking tablets regularly once or twice a day, and going to the doctor or nurse for check-ups every 3 months, are changes in behaviour. Each addition to the list adds to the risk of non-compliance or drop-out. Non-compliance will be selective, and patients may well choose to put effort into salt restriction, for which there is only contradictory evidence of small benefit, rather than stopping smoking, the benefit of which is enormous and beyond reasonable doubt. Most important of all, salt restriction makes it more difficult to change diet in other more important and better validated ways; we found that in their search for tasty food, salt-restricted subjects increased their intake of fatty and fried foods.

Conclusion on sodium restriction

Apart from being yet another task that has to be done (specific verbal advice with written back-up, and feedback from initial and follow-up measurements of 24-h urine sodium), sodium restriction by an easy 20–25% is a reasonable and effective adjunct to medication. A slow, decremental approach will minimise difficulties for the patient; a target of <80 mmol/day by 6 months is reasonable. We do not offer this routinely to the patients attending our clinic, because we do not have the necessary staff time available. We do offer if to patients who seem resistant to medication or who are on angiotensin converting enzyme (ACE) inhibitor drugs.

DIETARY POTASSIUM

Hunter-gatherer hypertension-free societies which consume ten times less salt than industrialised societies also consume much more potassium, both in fruit and unboiled vegetables, and as a condiment prepared from wood ash. Controlled trials of added potassium (64 mmol additional potassium daily) have shown a significant reduction in blood pressure in normotensives in 2 weeks (Khaw & Thom 1982) MacGregor et al 1982 found a significant 4% fall in mean blood pressure after 4 weeks in a double- blind crossover trial, adding 60 mmol potassium daily.

The main normal dietary sources of potassium are fruit and vegetables, raw or cooked by some method other than boiling, which leaches out the potassium; steaming, pressure-cooking, or microwave all conserve potassium without adding fat (Henningsen et al 1983). Another possible source is KCl-based salt, which tastes very different from NaCl, but in Finland a mixed salt has been developed which is more readily acceptable, and helps to raise the k/Na ratio, which may be how this hypotensive effect operates.

It is important to note that, unlike sodium restriction, there is evidence for a primary preventive effect of raised potassium intake on normotensive populations.

OBESITY

Obesity is best measured as body mass index (BMI, also known as Quetelet's index):

BMI = weight in kilograms/height in metres squared

Desirable weight is BMI 20–25. Plotting mortality against BMI, there is a U-curve, with excess mortality for both the very fat and the very thin. The upswing of the U-curve on the fat side becomes steep around BMI 30. I regard BMI 26–29 as cosmetic, >30 as medical. Using that definition, 12% of the Glyncorrwg population over 20 years old is medically obese. To use BMI, height needs to be recorded routinely at least once at age 20 or over, at a point in the record where it can be found easily.

Blood pressure is positively associated with weight-for-height at all ages (Kannel 1980), and change in weight is associated with change in blood pressure at younger ages (Miall et al 1968). Death rates from all causes are higher for fat people, and risks are less in those who can control their weight. Obesity has a bigger effect on death rates in the young than in the old (Seitzer 1966); for people 10 kg (about 23 lb) or more overweight, death rates are 46% higher than average at ages 15–34, 30% at 35–49, and 18% at 50–65. Very fat people who survive over the age of 65 have an almost average life expectancy (though they may be very disabled); their obesity is particularly resistant to treatment, and so, as with other risk factors, it is sensible to concentrate effort on the young and middle-aged.

Does weight reduction work?

Review of six intervention studies in 1980 suggested that weight reduction in obese hypertensives by energy intake restriction lowers blood pressure, at a rate of 3 mmHg systolic and 2 mmHg diastolic per 1 kg lost, up to 10 kg (Amery et al 1980). None of these studies used randomised controls. Surprisingly and disappointingly, a larger and much more powerful study than any of these, with a 4 kg loss in treated mild hypertensives and a loss of only 0.8 kg in untreated controls, showed no difference in either systolic or diastolic pressure (Kannel & Sorlie 1975). Entry diastolic pressures were in the range 90–104 mmHg, mean 135/91 mmHg, and mean age was 47.

The most likely explanations of this unexpected result are firstly, that at 47 they were already too old for hypertension to be reversible by weight control (this would be consistent with studies of Miall et al. (1968)); and secondly, that, as in sodium restriction, effects of weight reduction are greater in more severe hypertension, with a threshold around 170/100 mmHg.

Is it feasible?

Doctors tend to be nihilists about the treatment of obesity. Studies of consultations in which this was the principal diagnosis have shown that weight was measured and recorded in only about half, suggesting that at least half our GPs don't take treatment of obesity seriously. Pills are almost useless, so doctors trained to equate treatment with pill prescription quickly lose confidence. Opinion is often based on experience of giant obesity (BMI = >40), which is extremely difficult to treat even by specialists with full teaching hospital facilities. Such experience is irrelevant to control of obesity from a threshold of BMI 30.

Can it be harmful?

Like sodium restriction, control of obesity is yet another burden for patients. Unless there is a past or family history of medical obesity or maturity-onset diabetes, I think cosmetic obesity should be mentioned as a potential danger to be controlled, but otherwise left alone, unless the patient actually wants to lose weight and actively pursues this line of management. Anorectic drugs have little to commend them for anyone, and for hypertensives are contraindicated because they are likely to raise pressure.

For medical obesity, the most effective method of weight reduction seems to be a combination of diet and exercise, backed up by a specialised health worker (usually but not necessarily a dietitian), with initial personalised advice quickly moving to group work. When we reviewed all 80% or our treated hypertensives aged 40–64 in 1983, we found that 80% were above ideal weight, and one-third were medically obese (BMI >30).

We also compared the BMI available for 72 out of the original 98 hypertensives identified by screening our whole community in 1968 with their BMI in 1981 or at exit by death or moving away. Results are shown below:

Mean group BMI	1968–1969	1981 or exit
Men	29.7	27.6
Women	33.0	30.2
Both	31.0	28.6

These reductions were obtained in different ways for men and for women. The women have from time to time run weight-losing groups on a volunteer basis, with good results, but always eventually expiring from cumulative problems of leadership and organisation. We have learnt from experience that all self-help groups must be expected to have a beginning, a middle and an end. We had a male group going for about a year, led by an experienced dietitian. Long-term results were good, and many of these men have maintained good weight control ever since. The common assumption that only women are interested in or successful at weight control is wrong, but it is true that special effort is needed to set up male groups.

GLUCOSE INTOLERANCE

Figure 14.1 from the Framingham study (Kannel & Sorlie 1975), shows how the risk of cardiovascular disease increases by 60–80% with addition of glucose intolerance (not only frank diabetes) as a risk factor. Glucose intolerance is positively associated with high blood pressure and total blood cholesterol, as well as obesity and

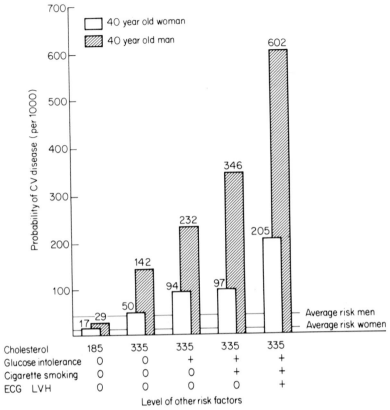

Fig. 14.1 Risk of cardiovascular (CV) diasease in 8 years at systolic blood pressure of 165 mmHg according to level of other risk factors. Framingham study: 18-year follow-up (Kannel & Sorlie 1975). (Reproduced with permission from: *Epidemiology and Control of Hypertension*, edited by P. Oglesby, Stratton Intercontinental, 1975).

hyperinsulinaemia. Most cases are reversible by control of obesity, and onset of frank diabetes can in many cases be prevented by weight control in first-degree relatives of diabetics (West 1978). Two-thirds of maturity-onset diabetics can regain normal glucose tolerance after 6 months of dietary treatment alone (Doar et al 1975).

ALCOHOL

This is a major problem in its own right, causing measurable liver damage, changes in peripheral blood or serious problems at work or in the home in about 12% of most adult male populations which have been thoroughly studied in Britain, and less than half that for women. It is an important cause of high blood pressure, is probably a precipitating factor for stroke, and is often linked with cigarette smoking. Routine search for alcohol problems in all patients, by taking a concise but specific alcohol history (how many drinks do you usually have on Mondays, Tuesdays, etc.) and by checking with the spouse, entering the result in an accessible part of a structured record, will greatly improve the quality and accuracy of care. Though the relation of alcohol to high blood pressure, coronary disease and stroke is certainly important, it is not yet sufficiently precise to be entered into a risk-equation.

Where the history or circumstantial evidence points to an alcohol problem, MCV and Gamma GT may give useful supporting evidence, but neither is by itself either specific or always sensitive. MCV >95 is a fairly sensitive indicator, particularly with long-standing problems. It returns to normal after about 3 months when drinking is controlled. Gamma GT is usually sensitive in younger patients, but is often normal in severe, advanced, and very obvious alcoholics. With early alcohol problems it responds quickly to control. Both these biochemical indicators are very useful in informing and motivating the patient and providing feedback on achievement. Our experience is that younger patients, or those with only the beginnings of a serious problem, respond well to advice and discussion, providing it is backed up by evidence of this kind. Morning blood alcohol (in a fluoride container) is occasionally useful in confirming suspicions, but we rarely find it helpful to confront patients with obvious discrepancies between their stated intake and evidence of this kind.

REFERENCES

Amery A, Bulpitt C, Fagard R et al 1980 Does diet matter in hypertension? European Heart Journal 1:299

Andrews G, McMahon S W, Austin A et al 1982 Hypertension: comparison of drug and non-drug treatments. British Medical Journal 284:1523. See also correspondence from Johnston D and Steptoe A 1982 British Medical Journal 285:1046

Beard T C, Cooke H M, Gray W R et al 1982 Randomised controlled trial of a no-added sodium diet for mild hypertension. Lancet ii:455

Bull N L, Buss D H 1980 Contribution of foods to sodium intake. Proceedings of the Nutrition Society 39:30A

Cooper R, Van Horn L, Liu K et al 1984 A randomized trial on the effect of decreased dietary sodium intake on blood pressure in adolescents. Journal of Hypertension 2:361

DeSwiet M 1982 Blood pressure, sodium, and take-away food. Archives of Disease in Childhood 57:645

Doar J W H, Wilde C E, Thompson M E et al 1975 Influence of treatment with diet alone on oral glucose tolerance test and plasma sugar and insulin levels in patients with maturity-onset diabetes mellitus. Lancet i:1263

Hart J T 1985 British blood cholesterol values and the American consensus. British Medical Journal 291:673

Henningsen N, Larsson L, Nelson D 1983 Hypertension, potassium, and the kitchen. Lancet i:133

Kannel W B 1980 Host and environmental determinants of hypertension: perspective from the Framingham study. In: Kesteloot H, Joossens J (eds) Epidemiology of arterial blood pressure. Martinus Nijhof, The Hague, p 265

Kannel W B, Sorlie P 1975 Hypertension in Framingham. In: Paul O (ed) Epidemiology and control of hypertension. Stratton Intercontinental, New York, p 553

Khaw K T, Thom S 1982 Randomised double-blind crossover trial of potassium on blood pressure in normal subects. Lancet ii:1127

MacGregor G A 1983 Dietary sodium and potassium intake and blood pressure. Lancet i:750

MacGregor G A, Markandu N D, Best F E et al 1982 Double-blind randomised crossover trial of moderate sodium restriction in essential hypertension. Lancet i:351

MacGregor G A, Smith S J, Markandu N D et al 1982 Moderate potassium supplementation in essential hypertension. Lancet ii:567

Medical Research Council 1950 The rice diet in the treatment of hypertension. Lancet ii:509

Miall W E, Bell R A, Lovell H G 1968 Relation between change in blood pressure and weight. British Journal of Preventive and Social Medicine 22:73

Morgan T, Adam W, Gillies A et al 1978 Hypertension treated by salt restriction. Lancet i:227

Nissinen A, Pietinen P, Tuomilehto J et al 1982 Experiments with dietary intervention in hypertension control; implementation of the North Karelia salt project. In: Altura B M (ed) Symposium on dietary minerals and cardiovascular disease, Tokyo 1982. Karger, Basel, p 232

Oliver M F 1983 Should we not forget about mass control of coronary risk factors? Lancet ii:37 and subsequent correspondence

Parfrey P S, Markandu N D, Roulston J E et al 1981 Relation between arterial pressure, dietary sodium intake, and renin system in essential hypertension. British Medical Journal 283:94

Puska P, Iacono J M, Nissinen A et al 1983 Controlled, randomised trial of the effect of dietary fat on blood pressure. Lancet i:1

Seltzer C C 1966 Some re-evaluations of the build and blood pressure study 1959 as related to ponderal index, somatotype and mortality. New England Journal of Medicine 274:254

Silman A J, Locke C, Mitchell P et al 1983 Evaluation of the effectiveness of a low sodium diet in the treatment of mild to moderate hypertension. Lancet i:1179

Watt G C M, Edwards C, Hart J T et al 1983 Dietary sodium restriction for mild hypertension in general practice. British Medical Journal 286:432. See also Watt G C M, Hart J T, Foy C J 1983 Effect of moderate dietary sodium restriction on patients with mild hypertension in general practice. Journal of Hypertension 1:18

West K M 1978 Epidemiology of diabetes. Elsevier, New York

15

Treatment without drugs: blood lipids, smoking, exercise and relaxation

The results of the MRC mild hypertension trial have finally confirmed what we already knew from other controlled trials; treatment of hypertension as an isolated risk factor is almost completely ineffective in reducing its most frequent lethal outcomes, coronary thrombosis and sudden heart death. Control of the two other principal risk factors, high blood cholesterol and smoking, are as important as reduction of blood pressure in the management of hypertension, and at pressures below about 175/105 mmHg, far more so.

BLOOD CHOLESTEROL, CORONARY DISEASE AND STROKE

A strong causal association between coronary heart disease and high total blood cholesterol, and a weaker link with stroke, are generally accepted. The main determinant of blood cholesterol is dietary fat.

Numerous studies in many countries have confirmed that blood cholesterol contributes little to stroke risk at any age, and cigarette smoking is also much less important than it is for coronary disease. As far back as records go — certainly long before any effective treatment for hypertension was available — stroke mortality has been falling in all countries with reliable statistics. The rate of decline of stroke mortality has speeded up since antihypertensive drugs have been available. There has also been a relative increase in the proportion of strokes attributed to thrombosis and embolism, and a decline in the proportion attributed to haemorrhage, suggesting that more severe hypertension is being effectively treated.

In Britain this fall in stroke mortality has coincided with the appearance for the first time of a gap between the stroke mortality of social classes I and II, and classes IV and V in the 1960 census, and has been increasing ever since. The difference was demon-

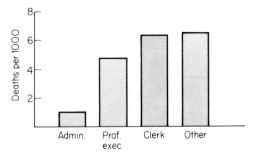

Fig. 15.1 Percentage of men in Whitehall study dying from stroke in 10 years (age-adjusted) according to grade of employment (Marmot et al 1978). (Reproduced with permission from: *The Journal of Epidemiology and Community Health*).

strated well in the Whitehall study of government employees, illustrated in Figure 15.1 (Marmot et al 1978). This gap may in part be caused by better delivery of antihypertensive treatment to people with higher and better informed expectations.

In contrast to stroke mortality, mortality from coronary disease and sudden heart death continued to rise until about 1973, and since then has stayed the same. Until the late 1960s, the USA had much higher coronary mortality rates than Britain, but a fall began in the USA around 1968, and between then and 1981 coronary mortality rates fell by 25–30%, so that US rates are now slightly lower than ours. These trends are shown in Figure 15.2 (Dwyer & Hetzel 1980).

The reasons for this fall are not fully understood (nor are all the causes of coronary heart disease), but changes in dietary fat are more consistent than falls in smoking (coronary mortality has fallen in US women as well as men, although women were smoking more and more throughout this period, while male smoking declined), and there is no convincing evidence that treatment of hypertension had any major impact. The absence of dietary change in Britain is the most likely explanation for our failure so far to follow this trend.

British GPs have been slow to act on blood cholesterol, and I have been among the slowest, despite being reasonably well informed of the causal link since the early 1960s. The reason for this is probably a fairly general reluctance to start a huge undertaking with (so most of us imagined) little chance of success. Properly organised prescription of antihypertensive drugs seemed an

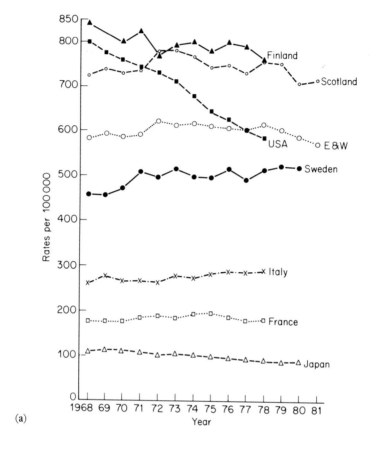

(a)

Fig. 15.2 Age-standardised ischaemic heart disease mortality rates in (a) men and (b) women aged 35–74 per 100 000. Data are given for the USA, England and Wales (E & W), Scotland, Finland, Sweden, Italy, France and Japan, for the period 1968 to 1981 (Marmor 1984).

easier and more readily defined task, more consistent with the nature of our training, which encouraged pharmacological intervention rather than responsibility for education to change behaviour.

Three development have begun to change this defeatist attitude. The first is the dramatic fall in US and Australian coronary death rates already referred to. The second is the now overwhelming evidence that, of the three classical coronary risk factors (blood pressure, smoking and cholesterol), cholesterol is the most important. The low coronary death rates in Japan and among black South Africans, who smoke heavily and have much severe hyper-

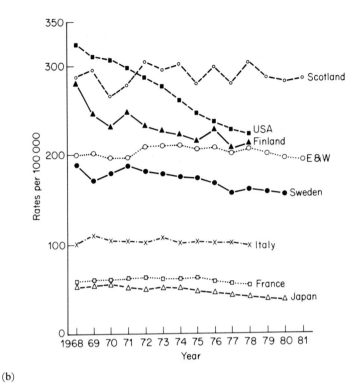

(b)

tension and high lung cancer and stroke mortality rates, but nearly all of whom have total blood cholesterols below 5 mmol (200 mg)/dl, are compelling evidence that of these three risk factors, only blood cholesterol is both a necessary and a sufficient cause. If total cholesterol is below 5 mmol/dl, it seems that neither blood pressure nor smoking cause coronary heart disease, though they still cause other kinds of fatal organ damage.

DIETARY FAT AND VEGETARIAN DIET

The third reason is the increasing evidence of the feasibility of reducing dietary saturated fat, and of its effectiveness in lowering blood pressure (Iacono et al 1975; Puska et al 1983; Rouse et al 1983) as well as reducing coronary heart mortality. Analysis of all controlled trials of blood cholesterol reduction before the Lipid Research Clinics trial shows that a 10% reduction in total cholesterol, whether achieved by drugs, diet or both, is associated with a roughly 20% reduction in subsequent coronary mortality (Peto 1985). Evidence that polyunsaturated fatty acids in fish oils reduce coronary mortality is also convincing (Kromhout et al 1985). There is now compelling evidence of the effectiveness of a high residue diet, low in sugar and saturated fat, in preventing or controlling a wide range of disorders from diverticulitis and diabetes to coronary disease and hypertension, vindicating in a remarkable way the original views of Cleave (1974).

The blood pressure-lowering effect of vegetarian diet is independent of fall in body weight (Puska et al 1983), and may be connected with the known blood pressure-lowering effect of increased dietary potassium discussed in Chapter 14.

WHAT SHOULD WE DO ABOUT CHOLESTEROL?

Anyone with a blood pressure high enough even to be considered for antihypertensive treatment is at greatly increased risk of coronary heart disease. Assessment of the other principal risk factors (family history, smoking and blood cholesterol) is important both in assessing risk, and in motivating the patient and the team. The first two are easy: all you have to do is ask, but (like blood pressure) nothing can be known about blood cholesterol unless you measure it. An initial measurement should be regarded as essential for every hypertensive patient.

What sort of measurement? Total cholesterol can be measured reliably on a non-fasting sample of clotted blood, and is stable for several days. HDL cholesterol is still more difficult to measure accurately, is usually thought to require a fasting sample, and there is some doubt whether it improves the predictive power of the measurement, at least in British populations (Pocock et al 1986), though this view is controversial.

Who needs treatment and follow-up? Roughly 80% of British adults have total cholesterol values over 5 mmol (200 mg)/dl, and would probably benefit from dietary advice. It is difficult to understand the logic of confining attention to those at highest risk, above say 7 mmol/dl total cholesterol; we don't do this with smoking, why do it with cholesterol? Of course, this would not be true for prescription of cholesterol-lowering drugs (see below), but these are rarely needed.

What advice should be given? This seems to be relatively simple, depending on five steps:

1. Reduce energy intake with the aim of attaining weight for height <BMI 30 for the frankly obese and <BMI 27 for those with cosmetic obesity.
2. Increase energy throughput by taking regular exercise.
3. Reduce fats of all kinds by one-quarter.
4. So far as possible, replace dairy and meat fats by vegetable and fish oils.
5. Increase vegetables and fruit, particularly those eaten raw, eat wholemeal bread, and increase the proportion of bread in the diet.

Follow-up measurements of cholesterol are important for feedback to people who undertake dietary change seriously. There is no need for measurements to be frequent or at standardised intervals, but evidence of success is the main incentive to carry on with what may initially be irksome restrictions.

There seems to me to be little place for cholesterol-lowering drugs, except in specialised clinics dealing with rare cases of hereditary hypercholesterolaemia. Clofibrate roughly doubles the incidence of symptomatic gallstones, and cholestyramine is both expensive and unpleasant.

SMOKING

Cigarettes raise blood pressure a little during the act of smoking, but otherwise smokers generally have slightly lower blood pressures than non-smokers, probably because they eat less and are generally a bit thinner. Patients and many nurses often believe the reason hypertensives should not smoke is that smoking raises blood pressure, and stopping smoking makes blood pressure fall. This belief can lead to disappointment and loss of compliance, so it is important to explain the independent effect of smoking on coronary risk, particularly in younger patients in whom this effect is most powerful; nearly all coronary deaths under 45 years of age are associated with smoking.

Smoking in treated hypertensives doubles their mortality (Bulpitt et al 1986), a memorable figure of which every hypertensive patient should be informed.

Is stopping smoking effective?

Doctors who quit smoking halved their mortality after 10 years, and most of this effect was apparent after the first year (Doll et al 1976), another simple figure which all hypertensives should know.

Is it feasible?

The beautiful controlled study of effectiveness of structured GP counselling for smokers in Australia reported in 1986 (Richmond et al) has now established beyond doubt the effectiveness of GP advice if we take this work seriously. At follow-up 3 years later, 35 of 100 smokers offered counselling had become and remained non-smokers, compared with 8 out of 100 controls not offered counselling. Patients were offered six consultations over 6 months, with discussion of personal risk profiles and review of the effects of smoking on patients' own peak expiratory flow rates.

British GPs are only beginning to take this work seriously, giving it the priority it deserves compared with other more traditional but much less effective work. Studies of medical records in teaching practices have shown the proportion of records containing any information about smoking habit to start from around 15–20% (Fleming & Lawrence 1981), though practices determined to change this achieve levels of 60% or more within a year.

Cost benefits for medical services from smoking control

Control of smoking is one of the few preventive measures likely to reduce both workload and treatment costs for primary care teams and hospitals, after only a few years. Study of a sample of 32 000 people in Exeter (Ashford 1973) showed that male smokers under the age of 45 had 33% more GP consultations, 47% more home visits, 26% more hospital outpatient consultations and 71% more inpatient days than non-smokers. Over the age of 45, care of smokers seems to shift toward hospitals, perhaps reflecting the seriousness of the diseases to which they are prone, with below average primary care workload but a 35% increase in hospital inpatient days.

EXERCISE

There is much fairly consistent evidence that regular exercise has a slight direct blood pressure-lowering effect, but changes are small and do not in themselves justify exercise programmes for hypertensives. Far more important is the more general effect on all forms of risk-taking behaviour; smoking, overeating, and the general state of health-unconsciousness from which regular exercise so often represents arousal. There is good evidence that men who take regular exercise are thinner, smoke less, have lower blood cholesterols and lower blood pressures than men who don't (Hickey et al 1975). People who reintroduce regular exercise to their lives, often for the first time since adolescence, generally enjoy life more, and adopt more positive attitudes to modifying their lives in other ways.

GPs can influence participation in exercise in the communities they serve providing they make a serious effort to do so (Campbell et al 1985). Availability of facilities for swimming and jogging should be known for your practice area. In working class areas particularly, facilities are often grossly deficient, and you should consider what can be done to improve matters. Local and even central government authorities are often responsive to pressure from medical groups, particularly if you can show the number of people potentially involved. The present Government's proposal that schools which own their full quota of green land should sell off one-third of it is a retreat from civilisation which could be successfully resisted if GPs were to act in supprot of the communities they serve.

Can it be harmful?

Advice to start slowly is important, particularly in obese and over-50s. Static exercise like press-ups and weight-lifting should be discouraged; it causes high peaks of blood pressure which can certainly be dangerous.

ENVIRONMENTAL STRESS

Fairly detailed knowledge of stresses at work (or out of it) and in the family are essential to good management, and may sometimes suggest individual causation. They are not usefully classifiable or measurable, and therefore cannot be used in calculating a risk-equation. There is now a very wide body of evidence suggesting that high coronary risk is related less to stress itself than to the socially determiend combination of high stress with powerlessness to do anything about it. Displacement by either promotion or demotion in the special pyramid, or by migration from a familiar culture to a new one, consistently raises coronary mortality rates in many studies.

Relaxation training

At an individual level, stress can be tackled either by helping patients to understand the nature of their powerlessness and thus in part to reduce it, or by helping them to adapt to it by learning a new set of physical responses. I know of no formal studies of the first technique, though it has been the main line I have tried to follow in my own practice.

Individual teaching in relaxation techniques has been developed and evaluated by controlled trial in several centres, notably by Chandra Patel. In a randomised controlled trial she has been able to show significant reductions in blood pressure persisting for 4 years after an initial training period (Patel et al 1985), as well as a significant reduction in ischaemic events. Her technique depends on a combination of teaching, practice and feedback, given at eight weekly 1-h sessions, run jointly by a nurse and a doctor, to patients in groups of ten. Her treatment plan is given in Appendix VII.

REFERENCES

Ashford J R 1973 Smoking and the use of health services. British Journal of Preventive and Social Medicine 27:8

Bulpitt C J, Beevers D G, Butler A et al 1986 The survival of treated hypertensive patients and their causes of death: a report from the DHSS Hypertensive Care Computing Project (DHCCP). Journal of Hypertension 4:93

Campbell M J, Browne D, Waters W E 1985 Can general practitioners influence exercise habits? British Medical Journal 290:1044

Cleave T L 1974 The saccharine disease. Wright, Bristol

Doll W R S, Peto R 1976 Mortality in relation to smoking: 20 years' observations on male British doctors. British Medical Journal 2:1525

Fleming D M, Lawrence M S T A 1981 An evaluation of recorded information about preventive measures in 38 practices. Journal of the Royal College of General Practitioners 31:615

Hickey N, Mulcahy R, Bourke G J et al 1975 Study of coronary risk factors related to physical activity in 15 171 men. British Medical Journal iii:507

Iacono J M, Marshall M W, Dougherty R M et al 1975 Reduction in blood pressure associated with high polyunsaturated fat diets that reduce blood cholesterol in man. Preventive Medicine 4:426

Kannel W B, Dawber T R, Kagan A, Revotskie N, Stokes J 1961 Factors of risk in the development of coronary heart disease: six-year follow-up experience in the Framingham study. Annals of Internal Medicine 55:33

Kromhout D, Bosschieter E B, Coulander C L 1985 The inverse relation between fish consumption and 20-year mortality from coronary heart disease. New England Journal of Medicine 312:1205

Marmot M G 1984 Lifestyle and national and international trends in coronary heart disease mortality. Postgraduate Medical Journal 60:3

Marmot M G, Rose G, Shipley M et al 1978 Employment grade and coronary heart disease in British civil servants. Journal of Epidemiology and Community Health 32:244

Patel C, Marmot M G, Terry D J et al 1985 Trial of relaxation in reducing coronary risk: four year follow up. British Medical Journal 290:1103

Peto R 1985 Contribution to discussion. In: Evered D, Whelan J (eds) The value of preventive medicine (Ciba Foundation symposium 110). Pitman, London, p 77

Pocock S J, Shaper A G, Phillips A N et al 1986 High density lipoprotein cholesterol is not a major risk factor for ischaemic heart disease in British men. British Medical Journal 292:515

Puska P, Nissinen A, Vartiainen E et al 1983 Controlled, randomised trial of the effect of dietary fat on blood pressure. Lancet i:1

Richmond R L, Austin A, Webster I W 1986 Three year evaluation of a programme by general practitioners to help patients to stop smoking. British Medical Journal 292:803

Rouse J L, Beilin L J, Armstrong B K et al 1983 Blood pressure-lowering effect of a vegetarian diet: controlled trial in normotensive subjects. Lancet i:5

16

Antihypertensive drugs in general

All effective drugs have potential for harm as well as good, and because the absolute reduction of risk is generally small in patients without evidence of organ damage even over periods of several years, cumulative risks over several decades of treatment may easily exceed benefits unless patients and drugs are both selected carefully, and there is a permanent state of alertness for side-effects, interactions and unnecessary treatment. In the absence of acute heart failure, brain damage, or retinal haemorrhage or oedema, the decision to start antihypertensive treatment should only be made after at least three and preferably more readings of blood pressure. Initial choice of drug should include methodical review of potential risks in that particular patient, and initial baseline measurements should be made of any variables likely to be affected by medication.

THE HISTORICAL SEQUENCE

From time to time suggestions are made for a more or less standard sequence of drugs to be used as an optimal treatment plan (stepped care). These suggestions may be practicable in a hospital outpatient setting or a hitherto untreated population, where there is a steady inward flow of new cases to whom a standard treatment protocol can be applied, but they are of little use for the care of populations with an established tradition of GP care. The primary care team inherits a population much of which is already receiving a ragbag of antihypertensive drugs, reflecting the medications in vogue when each patient started treatment, as well as the different prescribing habits of previous doctors. Even among contemporaries it is usually difficult to agree on a standard sequence of drug groups, or on choices of particular drugs within groups. One of the most difficult but necessary steps in antihypertensive care is to get patients to take medication regularly; anything likely to disturb a nicely established pattern is rightly viewed with suspicion, so that otherwise obsolete drugs which are well tolerated and seem to be doing a good job may continue in use for 20 or 30 years, disrupting currently recommended patterns of prescribing.

Ganglionic and preganglionic blocking drugs such as bethanidine and guanethidine, though very effective in controlling pressure, cause disabling side-effects and no longer have a place in routine treatment. Some other older drugs, however, have been prematurely discarded. It is worth bearing in mind that the older drugs were all initially used in excessive dosage in (by hindsight) often unrealistic attempts to obtain control with a single agent, thus giving them a sometimes undeserved reputation for toxicity. This applies particularly to reserpine, which has almost gone out of use though in low dosage it is a safe, usually well tolerated, effective, and extremely cheap drug. There is little profit in the older drugs, so they are no longer promoted, and tend to be used only by older doctors (like me). Their long history ensures that we already have most of the bad news about their long-term side-effects, in contrast to newer and necessarily relatively untried drugs.

EFFECTS ON OTHER RISK FACTORS

Because all hypertensives are at greatly increased risk for coronary heart disease, and because control of blood pressure has so far had very disappointing results in reducing this risk, beneficial or adverse effects of antihypertensive drugs on other major coronary risk factors should be an important consideration in selecting medication. Thiazide diuretics are particularly suspect in this respect, having small but probably significant adverse effects on glucose tolerance and total blood cholesterol, which increase with age and duration of treatment. Beta-blockers also probably have a small adverse effect on total blood cholesterol. Prazosin, on the other hand, seems to have quite a large favourable effect on total cholesterol.

EVIDENCE ON IATROGENIC IMPAIRMENT

Impairments and risks associated with individual antihypertensive drugs are discussed fully in Chapter 17. A study in general practice by Jachuk et al (1982) showed that in 75 controlled hypertensives none of their GPs was aware of any impairments associated with treatment, but 10% of patients admitted to adverse effects on direct questioning, and when the same question was asked of close relatives and workmates, they reported adverse effects in 74% (mild in 25%, moderate in 45%, and severe in 30%). Doctors are insensitive to impairments caused by drugs they have prescribed, particularly if (as must often be the case) symptoms are non-specific (fatigue, minor depression, loss of appetite or interest) or of a private nature (impotence or loss of libido). This can be said with confidence, because though doctors all over the world were prescribing thiazide diuretics on a colossal scale ever since these useful drugs came on the market in the late 1950s, the first report of a single case of impotence associated with their use appeared only in 1977, and even this was generally overlooked until 1981, when the MRC trial revealed that after 1 year's treatment impotence was found in 10% of men on placebo treatment, 13% on propranolol and 23% on thiazides (MRC 1981). Evidently, we didn't want to know.

DRUG AND DISEASE INTERACTIONS

Antihypertensive treatment on a mass scale is directed mainly at people in middle and old age, liable to a host of other ailments which also need treatment. Patients are aware of the possibilities of drug interactions, and unless you discuss these with them, may think they must choose between different medications themselves for fear of precipitating chemical quarrels in their insides, or construct impossibly complex treatment timetables to avoid encounters between incompatible pills.

The most important and most frequently overlooked interaction with all antihypertensive drugs is with indomethacin and other non-steroidal anti-inflammatory agents (NSAIDs) operating through prostaglandin-synthetase inhibition. Indomethacin increases blood pressure by about 19/9 mmHg in patients on diuretics or beta-blockers (Watkins et al 1980), almost completely eliminating their hypotensive effect. It is pointless to use NSAIDs for painful but non-inflammatory joint conditions like degenerative arthrosis and backache other than ankylosing spondylitis, so part of the answer is to use these drugs only when they are truly necessary. Now that many of them are available from pharmacies without prescription, it is important to ask patients if they are taking them for headaches, joint pain, or general aches.

Cimetidine is another commonly prescribed long-term treatment, which increases bioavailability of metoprolol and propranolol; there is no effect on atenolol (Kirch et al 1981).

Though nifedipine can be safely combined with beta-blockers, and this combination has been used on a mass scale, it can occasionally precipitate heart failure.

Clonidine, a centrally acting drug now little-used, is more likely than other antihypertensive drugs to produce dangerous rebound hypertension if the drug is stopped or one or two doses are omitted, if used with beta-blockers or tricyclic antidepressants. The wisest policy is probably not to use it at all.

The effect of antidiabetic agents is opposed by thiazide diuretics, though the combination is not absolutely contraindicated. All beta-blockers mask the warning symptoms of hypoglycaemia, so they can be dangerous in unstable diabetics. They have little effect on blood sugar control or glucose tolerance. In patients with liver damage they may have a positive advantage, by lowering portal vein pressure and thereby possibly making bleeding from oesophageal varices less likely.

Though not strictly a drug interaction, compatibility of all antihypertensive drugs with moderate quantities of alcohol should be discussed with patients — otherwise they are likely to stop their medication every weekend.

There are no important interactions between any commonly used antihypertensive drugs and drugs used for control of epilepsy or airways obstruction.

CHOOSING AND CHANGING ANTIHYPERTENSIVE DRUGS

Within the main groups of antihypertensive drugs, it is important to agree within your team on one or at most two individual drugs, and stick to them so that what must at best be a confused situation does not become totally incomprehensible. Try also to agree on both generic prescribing and generic recording and discussion. There are already 50 different generic drugs listed in the British National Formulary approved for use as antihypertensive agents; is it really possible to think at all about what you are doing, if you add another 150 brand names?

FOUR RULES FOR STARTING, STOPPING AND CHANGING

In the Glyncorrwg clinic, we have found the following four rules useful:

Rule 1: Start and stop slowly

Nearly all side-effects are dose-dependent. Unless you start with the smallest possible dose, you will not find the fortunate minority of patients who respond exceptionally easily, and may saddle them with a lifetime of unnecessary risk. Start slowly, and add increments at weekly or monthly intervals until you either have control, or are forced to add another antihypertensive drug.

Methyldopa, beta-blockers and clonidine can all cause severe rebound hypertension if they are stopped abruptly. Unless they are causing a serious side-effect, all of them should be stopped decrementally over 2 or 3 days, and except for diuretics (which are only given in low dosage anyway) it seems wise to apply this rule to all antihypertensive medication, and stop slowly.

Rule 2: Make all decisions on more than one reading

If you unexpectedly get one high reading, don't immediately raise the dose or add another drug; think about possible causes (missed tablets, rushing to the surgery, a full bladder, a very cold day) and get one or two more readings over the next day or two, before changing treatment.

Rule 3: Don't add new drugs unless you really need to

Few patients really need more than two antihypertensive drugs. When you find yourself thinking about a third drug (which may be the fifth, sixth, or seventh in a patient with other long-term problems such as chronic airways obstruction, arthritis, duodenal ulcer or diabetes) check through other possible causes of failure; unchallenged obesity, heavy alcohol intake, or systematic non-compliance with treatment already prescribed.

Rule 4: Change one drug at a time

If you change more than one drug at a time, there is no way of identifying the real source of changes, either adverse or beneficial. This means that fixed dose combinations, which may be very useful once the patient has settled down on effective medication, should never be used at the start. High prescription charges make this sensible policy difficult to implement.

RELATIVE COSTS

Sooner or later, GPs and their teams are likely to become local budget-holders in the NHS. A patient taking bendrofluazide 2.5 mg twice a day costs the nation £2.99 a year (at 1986 prices, here and subsequently, and ignoring prescription charges). If a second drug is required, you might add reserpine, which as one combined tablet twice a day would cost only £3.91 a year. If you were worried about cholesterol levels, you might choose prazosin 2 mg twice a day, which together with bendrofluazide would raise the cost to £53.94 a year. Finally, if nothing worked except an ACE blocker, enalapril 20 mg a day plus a thiazide would cost £344.63 a year.

In the Third World, these differences are really important. In practice, continuing treatment for hypertension is almost entirely restricted to a tiny minority of wealthy patients, who often tend to be treated with whatever is the latest, most heavily promoted, and most expensive drug. Attending a conference on control of hypertension in the community in Bogotá in 1984, I found that neither generic thiazides nor reserpine of any kind were available anywhere in Colombia, and that physicians prescribing enough of more profitable drugs were rewarded with a free Volkswagen by grateful pharmaceutical companies.

REFERENCES

Jachuk S J, Brierley H, Jachuk S et al 1982 The effect of hypotensive drugs on the quality of life. Journal of the Royal College of General Practitioners 32:103
Kirch W, Kohler H, Spahn H et al 1981 Interaction of cimetidine with metoprolol, propranolol, or atenolol. Lancet ii:531
Medical Research Council Working Party 1981 Adverse reactions to bendrofluazide and propanolol for the treatment of mild hypertension. Lancet ii:539
Watkins J, Abbott E C, Hensby C N et al 1980 Attenuation of hypotensive effect of propranolol and thiazide diuretics by indomethacin. British Medical Journal 281:702

17

Individual antihypertensive drugs

The historical order in which the main drugs now in use have been introduced is as follows (year of first marketing in brackets):

Reserpine	(1949)
Hydralazine	(1951)
Diuretics	(1957)
Methyldopa	(1963)
Clonidine	(1966)
Beta-blockers	(1966)
Prazosin	(1976)
Calcium blockers	(1979)
ACE inhibitors	(1981)

They are discussed in that order in this chapter.

RESERPINE

Reserpine came into general use in the 1950s, more or less simultaneously with thiazide diuretics, and these two together were the principal drugs used for treatment of all but the most severe cases of high blood pressure for about 20 years, including the Veterans Administration trials on which all thoughtful policies were based up to the late 1970s. Reserpine's antihypertensive effect operates through depletion of catecholamines in the brainstem, and the high doses originally used were a common cause of severe depression, which was sometimes suicidal. This, together with more profitable and vigorously promoted alternatives, led to its virtual extinction from British practice, though it lingered on in the USA where introduction of beta-blockers was delayed by more cautious legislation.

Reserpine is a cheap and effective drug when used in small doses with a thiazide diuretic; it is more effective in fact than the combination diuretic plus beta-blocker (Veterans Administration

1977). Provided that dosage starts at 0.05 mg and a maximum dosage of 0.3 mg daily is not exceeded, incidence of depression is no higher than with other commonly used antihypertensive drugs (McMahon 1978; Veterans Administration 1982). It is particularly useful for cases resistant to other drugs; these often show a dramatic response to addition of a small dose of reserpine. It has a slow, prolonged effect, which may take several weeks to wear off when the drug is stopped, and is fully effective in once-daily dosage.

Neither this nor any other centrally acting antihypertensive drug (methyldopa, clonidine, propranolol and other lipid-soluble beta-blockers) should be used in patients who are already depressed, or in people with Parkinson's disease. A stuffed-up nose is a common side-effect. A slowed pulse is invariable (and a useful marker of compliance), so it should not be used in patients with heart block.

HYDRALAZINE

Hydralazine is another inheritance from the past, encountered occasionally in patients who started treatment in the 1960s, but rarely used for new cases. It was popular in the USA, but was never so widely used in Britain. It is an arteriolar vasodilator, rarely effective and poorly tolerated on its own, but forming a rational, effective, and usually well tolerated combination with beta-blockers. It can be given in twice-daily dosage.

The main problem with hydralazine is the development of lupus erythematosus (LE) syndrome in 10–20% of patients at doses over 200 mg daily (Bing et al 1980; Mansilla-Tinoco et al 1982), usually presenting with joint pains which are indistinguishable clinically from rheumatoid arthritis, sometimes with malaise and/or weight loss. The LE syndrome is fully though slowly reversible by stopping the drug. Dosage should never exceed 200 mg daily, but even then LE syndrome occurs in 1–3% of patients. Risk is much higher in slow-acetylators and in women. The test for acetylator status is simple to arrange, and should be done in anyone maintained on this drug (ring your local laboratory for details). Development of LE syndrome is usually preceded by a positive titre for antinuclear factor (ANF), but not all those with a positive ANF develop this complication, and it is not a good reason for stopping the drug if there is no clinical illness. LE syndrome usually develops months or years after starting hydralazine, and the most difficult problem is to remember, when it occurs, that joint pains may not be what they seem; more than one patient has been left on hydralazine, and started on long-term treatment for her 'rheumatoid arthritis'. Impotence is another fairly common and reversible side-effect.

DIURETICS

Diuretics were the first easily used and well tolerated antihypertensive drugs available, coming into general use in the late 1950s. Compared with the very potent but extremely unpleasant ganglion-blockers, and less powerful but more tolerable drugs like reserpine and hydralazine which preceded them, they seemed to be almost completely free from side-effects. This reputation has stuck, so the decision to use them is often made casually, and when side-effects do occur they are often ignored or blamed on another drug.

Diuretics are generally rather more effective in lowering blood pressure than (for example) beta-blockers, but they often cause troublesome symptoms and have some worrying long-term side-effects. However, they do have two very great advantages; they are extremely cheap, and their very long track record means that at least we already have most of the bad news about them. Like many other antihypertensive drugs, we are still unsure how they work; some of their effect may be through sodium depletion, but they also have a vasodilator effect.

It is now at last generally understood that diuretics exert their full antihypertensive effect at low dosage, at which the risk of side-effects is minimal. There is no point in giving more than 2.5 mg twice a day of bendrofluazide, or 25 mg once a day of chlorthalidone. Thiazide diuretics have a much bigger antihypertensive effect than loop diuretics (for example, frusemide), and long-acting diuretics like chlorthalidone are more convenient than shorter-acting diuretics like bendrofluazide, which must be given twice a day.

Patients are usually told they are 'water tablets', which can be helpful when trying to sort out a row of small unlabelled bottles containing various sizes of white pills. It is important to explain to patients that, although they do indeed promote the outflow of water, they have been prescribed to control blood pressure, not to increase urine output. If patients don't understand this, they may easily decide that since urine flow is all too free (particularly at night), there is no need to continue the tablets. Nocturia is not always caused by diuretics; nifedipine is also a frequent cause.

Diuretics are contraindicated in pregnancy because they reduce placental bloodflow.

Side-effects of diuretics

Diuretics have six important side-effects: tiredness and depression, erectile failure, gout, glucose intolerance, reduction in blood potassium, and raised blood cholesterol. Tiredness and depression, though rarely severe, are common side-effects of diuretics, as well as of all other antihypertensive drugs; you should ask about this at the first follow-up visit after starting. Though diuretics are often (and correctly) used in fixed combination with other antihypertensive drugs, they should never be started this way, because then it is impossible to decide which drug in the combination is responsible for any side-effects.

Erectile failure in men is common, affecting 16% of men after 12 weeks of treatment in the MRC trial (1981). You should mention this possibility to men when starting the drug, together with the MRC figure, which helps to put the risk in reasonable perspective. The effect is quickly reversible when the drug is stopped. Other antihypertensive drugs also cause impotence occasionally, generally at less than a quarter of this rate. Erectile failure is in any case common in hypertensives and particularly in diabetics, usually because of atheroma in the arteries supplying the penis, or ischaemic nerve damage; failure from this cause is much less likely to improve. This possibility should be explained to patients who do develop erectile failure while on diuretics; otherwise the drug may be blamed incorrectly for permanent impotence. Don't be afraid to talk about this; I have never yet met a patient who resented such an enquiry, but men who may for years have attributed their impotence to their hypertension rather than its treatment have every right to resent failure to give them accurate information. No research studies appear to have been done on the effects of diuretics on sexual function in women.

Gout is a common outcome of long-term treatment with diuretics, which nearly always raises blood urate levels. Again, the effect is reversible. Glucose intolerance is more important, since diabetes is a very important risk factor for coronary disease and stroke, but it is said to be unlikely that drug-induced glucose intolerance has the same harmful effect as naturally occurring diabetes (Jarrett 1983). It tends to develop after 2 or 3 years of treatment, and is much commoner in the elderly (Murphy et al

1982). The attack rate for frank diabetes was about 9 per 1000 patient-years of treatment in the MRC trial, and in 40% of cases glucose tolerance remained abnormal despite withdrawal of the drug. It is usually unwise to start treatment with diuretics in subjects who are seriously overweight or have a family history of diabetes, and diuretics should be avoided if possible in patients who already have diabetes. Because assiduous control of raised blood pressure slows decline in renal function in diabetics, the choice sometimes has to be made; there can be no doubt at all that diuretics do more good than harm to diabetics, if hypertension cannot be controlled otherwise.

The rise in blood cholesterol with prolonged use of diuretics is worrying because, like glucose intolerance, it increases the risk of coronary disease. Some studies have suggested a large effect (Grimm et al 1981). In the MRC trial (1985) cholesterols rose by less than 1% after 3 years on thiazides, but as those on placebo had a 2% fall in cholesterol, the true rise could be around 3%. This doesn't sound much, but applied to several million hypertensives already at high risk it must cause some deaths.

Again in the MRC trial (1985), mean blood potassium levels fell from an initial 4.1 to 3.6 mmol after 3 years, compared with a rise from 4.1 to 4.2 mmol on placebo. However, there is little evidence that diuretics in the small doses which should be used for anti-hypertensive treatment increase the number of ectopic heartbeats or the frequency of serious arrhythmias, even in elderly patients (Coope 1983). Even the most carefully formulated slow-release forms of potassium supplement, whether given alone or in fixed combination with diuretics, do produce some mucosal gut damage in most young and healthy experimental volunteers (McMahon et al 1982), so it seems that more harm than good is probably done by routine potassium supplements of any kind in the diuretic treatment of high blood pressure.

Provided that baseline electrolytes are measured before starting treatment, the safest policy is probably simply to remain alert for the possibility that complaints of weakness may be caused by hypokalaemia. Serious hypokalaemia is extremely unlikely in patients with uncomplicated hypertension who are otherwise well, and is unusual even in the presence of heart failure (Morgan & Davidson 1980; Sandor et al 1982). Risks are greatly increased in patients also receiving digoxin.

An alternative where there is a high risk of hypokalaemia is to choose one of the potassium-sparing diuretics: amiloride, triamterene or spironolactone. Amiloride and triamterene are almost always used in fixed combination with a low dose of thiazide, though amiloride alone with a beta-blocker is apparently just as effective in controlling blood pressure as thiazide alone with a beta-blocker (Thomas & Thomson 1983). Triamterene commonly causes granular casts, suggesting at least some renal damage, though there is no evidence of impaired function (Fairley et al 1983). The aldosterone antagonist spironolactone, first introduced in 1960, has little effect on blood pressure alone (except in hyperaldosteronism however caused), but used in combination with a thiazide has a substantial blood pressure-lowering effect, while conserving potassium. This is expensive, rarely necessary, and can get you in deep trouble if the patient goes into renal failure with potassium retention, or if someone inadvertently prescribes potassium supplements. This can happen very easily in the often confused medication of the elderly.

METHYLDOPA

Methyldopa was introduced in 1963 and rapidly came into wide use. Patients who started it then are now in their 70s, so it is still much used in the elderly.

Methyldopa remains the principal drug used for hypertension in pregnancy (de Swiet 1985), although it crosses the placental barrier. It is probably slightly more effective in controlling pressure than beta-blockers, and there is little difference in maternal or fetal outcome (Fidler et al 1983). Any substantial permanent impairment in later brain function in the child has been excluded (Ounsted et al 1980), and any possible smaller effect must be balanced against the high rate of fetal loss and prematurity, as well as the danger to the mother, of untreated hypertension in pregnancy.

Like reserpine, Methyldopa acts centrally, probably by catecholamine depletion. It is effective in once-daily dosage, best given in the early evening because of its usually marked sedative effect, which lasts into the morning if it is given at bedtime. At doses over 500 mg/day it nearly always causes drowsiness, which can be a serious hazard, particularly in elderly car-drivers.

Methyldopa causes measurable liver damage in about 3% of patients (Hoyumpa & Connell 1973; Sataline & Lowell 1976), and should be avoided in heavy drinkers or anyone with a raised gamma GT or other impaired liver function tests, or with gallbladder disease. It is an occasional cause of cholestatic jaundice, which, because about 20% of all adults have radiologically demonstrable gallstones (usually without symptoms), may be very difficult to diagnose precisely.

Methyldopa interferes with many laboratory tests, causing misleading results unless you remember to mention its use on the request form. It interacts with major phenothiazines to produce a paradoxical increase in blood pressure, increases the toxicity of lithium, and disturbs treatment of Parkinson's disease with L-dopa. At doses under 1 g daily, about 10% of patients on methyldopa develop a positive direct Coomb's test (Carstairs et al 1966; Harth 1968), evidence of the first stage in an autoimmune process. About 2% of all patients go on to develop an autoimmune haemolytic anaemia, which is usually reversible if treatment is stopped promptly.

Except for its use in pregnancy, methyldopa is becoming obsolete, though I still use it because it is a devil I know and many patients are still happy with it. Because of common contraindications to beta-blockers, it is still occasionally necessary to start it in elderly patients with severe hypertension, though about a quarter of all patients have to stop methyldopa within 6 months because of adverse side-effects (Ramsay 1981). If you do use it in the elderly, baseline liver function tests should be recorded and compared with a follow-up measurement 3 to 6 months later.

CLONIDINE

Clonidine came into use in 1966. It was developed in the Federal Republic of Germany and is still very widely used there. It never became popular in the UK, in my opinion rightly so. It has both central and peripheral blocking actions on catecholamines, which cause depression and fatigue in about half of all patients, but its most serious disadvantage is that blocked catecholamines accumulate, and may be suddenly released if the drug is stopped, leading to severe rebound hypertension (Goldberg et al 1977; Reid et al 1977). Rebound hypertension is an occasional problem after sudden withdrawal of virtually all antihypertensive drugs other than thiazides and reserpine, but clonidine is in a class by itself in this respect.

BETA-BLOCKERS

Though in general beta-blockers impede the links between nervous inputs and vascular reactivity, their mode of action is still not fully understood. They reduce blood pressure slightly less than diuretics, though as with other antihypertensive drugs there is wide individual variability in response. The dose required for beta-blockade, as shown by a slow heart rate, is often less than that required for maximum reduction in pressure, and the full antihypertensive effect of beta-blockers may take 3 or 4 weeks to appear.

When beta-blockers were first introduced in the mid-1960s, there were high hopes that they might break the causal sequence widely assumed to be operating in essential hypertension — environmental stress + vulnerable personality → raised autonomic drive → raised blood pressure — so they were attractive as drugs operating on causes rather than modifying effects. Moreover they were competing with and rapidly replacing methyldopa, which was often given in a high dosage of 2 g/day or more. Compared with this, propranolol (the first beta-blocker) was well tolerated; life was transformed for many patients, just as it had been when methyldopa rescued hypertensives from the severe side-effects of ganglion-blockers.

There was also reasonable hope that beta-blockers might have a specific preventive effect on arrhythmias, preventing many sudden deaths from ischaemic heart disease; right up to the late 1970s, there was mounting but always inconclusive evidence that this might be so. Beta-blockers seemed to be specially effective in reducing the variability of blood pressure during the day, reducing alarm response as one would expect from their mode of action. Finally, beta-blockers prevented angina in the many hypertensives who had this symptom, so they were widely used for this purpose in patients with only borderline high blood pressure.

There was a brief interruption in their rapid spread when one cardioselective variant, practolol, was found to cause serious and irreversible autoimmune fibrosis of the conjunctiva, middle ear, pleura, pericardium and peritoneum (oculomucocutaneous syndrome), but this seems to have been unique to practolol. Suspicions that other beta-blockers may cause occasional cases of retroperitoneal fibrosis seem to be without foundation (Pryor et al 1983). Similar fears that they might cause Peyronie's disease (obstruction of the penile artery with fibrous plaques) have also proved groundless (Pryor & Castle 1982). The common assertion that intermittent claudication is worsened by beta-blockers is in my experience untrue, a view which is now supported by controlled studies (Bogaert & Crement 1983). There were also fears that beta-blockers would become a common cause of heart failure because they reduce heart output, but even in the elderly this seems to happen surprisingly rarely.

The hopes have not been realised in practice. The MRC trial of treatment for mild hypertension (1985) showed no cardioprotective advantage for beta-blockers in mild hypertension, and there is no reason to believe results would be any better in more severe hypertension. There is now fairly consistent evidence that beta-blockers are less effective in black than in white patients (Veterans Administration 1982). Though much better tolerated than methyldopa, beta-blockers now have to compete with prazosin, calcium channel blockers and ACE inhibitors.

Side-effects of beta-blockers

Beta-blockers slow the heart (a useful sign that the tablets are being taken) and reduce heart output. They should not be used in subjects who already have heart block or are in low-output heart failure.

All beta-blockers cause bronchoconstriction in patients with hyper-reactive airways. This may be severe and has caused death in asthmatics, and asthma should be regarded as an absolute contraindication to use of all beta-blockers. The effect is smaller with cardioselective beta-blockers, such as atenolol and metoprolol, than it is with unselective beta-blockers like propranolol, but it is not safe to use any of them in people with symptomatic asthma. No patient should ever be started on beta-blocker drugs without an initial measurement of PEFR, which should be compared with the expected PEFR for his or her age and height on the chart provided with the flowmeter. Such routine measurements reveal many unsuspected cases of reversible airways obstruction. If PEFR is 25% or more below the expected value, give a test inhalation of 400 μ salbutamol and repeat the measurement 20 minutes later; a 20% improvement is diagnostic of reversible airways obstruction.

In many patients with fairly severe airways obstruction, it is irreversible. Generally speaking, these patients are not adversely affected by beta-blockers, but even then PEFR should be monitored for the first five or six visits.

About one-third of patients on beta-blockers feel tired and lethargic or complain of muscle weakness (Bai et al 1982); in my experience this is a more serious problem in heavy manual workers than sedentary workers.

The MRC mild hypertension trial (1985) showed that in patients who continue to smoke, coronary mortality is actually higher in mild hypertensives treated with propranolol than in those treated only with a placebo. The reason for this is not clear, but the finding is consistent and cannot be disregarded. Beta-blockers as a group reduce the protective HDL fraction of blood cholesterol and increase triglyceride (Leren et al 1980; Berglund & Andersson 1981).

Because of their popularity over many years, many patients are now well controlled on beta-blockers which they tolerate well, but their use in new patients is likely to diminish rapidly as the lessons of the MRC trial sink in. A cardioprotective effect for 1 to 3 years after recovery from myocardial infarction has been clearly shown for propranolol and timolol, but results for sotalol and oxprenolol were equivocal, suggesting that this effect, which is still not fully understood, must be regarded as specific for these two drugs (Opie 1984).

Beta-blockers can be used in pregnancy without any more evidence of fetal damage than methyldopa (Fidler et al 1983), but they also cross the placental barrier and seem to be slightly less effective in controlling the mother's blood pressure.

Drug interaction with beta-blockers

Cimetidine greatly increases the bioavailability of propranolol and metoprolol (Donovan et al 1981; Kirch et al 1981). Atenolol seems to be unaffected.

Which beta-blocker? (Breckenridge 1983; Cameron & Ramsay 1983)

Ten different beta-blockers (including one alpha-beta-blocker) are marketed in Britain, as well as various fixed combinations with diuretics and slow-release formulations. The most lipid-soluble of these (propranolol, oxprenolol, metoprolol and timolol) are the most likely to enter the brain cells and cause central side-effects such as depression, tiredness and bad dreams. The most water-soluble variants (atenolol, nadolol and sotalol) on the other hand, are mainly excreted through the kidney and therefore accumulate in patients with renal damage. Although cardioselectivity is relative and no beta-blockers are safe in people with increased airways reactivity, the unselective beta-blockers like propranolol and nadolol are more dangerous, and their bronchoconstricting effects more difficult to reverse, than the most cardioselective beta-blockers atenolol, metoprolol, and acebutolol.

There seems to be little clinical difference between atenolol and metoprolol, both of which are cardioselective. Atenolol is effective in once-daily dosage, but metoprolol has a shorter halflife and should be given twice a day. Atenolol is not lipid-soluble, and this may make it less likely to cause central side-effects such as depression and bad dreams. Atenolol costs nearly three times as much as metoprolol in equivalent dosage, but for reasons known only to the companies concerned, the tablet combining atenolol with chlorthalidone costs only 40% more than the tablet combining metoprolol with hydrochlorothiazide. A slow-release form of metoprolol is available which can be given once a day, but this costs even more than atenolol.

The alpha-beta blocker labetalol seems to offer no advantage in practice over other variants, and is also expensive.

PRAZOSIN

This vasodilator was introduced in 1976, and has probably made hydralazine obsolete. It is a natural combination with beta-blockers, reducing the bradycardia and cold extremities which are otherwise often troublesome.

The greatest advantage of prazosin is that it reduces total blood cholesterol by about 9% and triglycerides by 16%, without any reduction in protective HDL lipoprotein (Leren et al 1980). This is a very substantial effect, greater than that achieved in most dietary control programmes. Used in combination with beta-blockers, prazosin almost but not quite cancels out the increase in blood cholesterol induced by beta-blockers.

The greatest disadvantage of prazosin is syncopal fainting with the first dose. To avoid this, the possibility should be explained, the first dose should be given at bedtime, and should be not more than 0.5 mg (half of a 1 mg scored tablet), building up to a maximum dose of 20 mg daily, though 4 mg is usually sufficient in combination with another antihypertensive drug. Faintness from postural hypotension remains a problem in about 14% of patients (Pitts 1974), and it is probably unwise to start it in elderly patients, or people who already have symptoms of vertebrobasilar insufficiency. Another common problem with prazosin used on its own is water retention, with oedema of the feet, but this is not a problem when prazosin is combined with a diuretic. Prazosin can be given in twice-daily dosage.

Prazosin is very effective in combination with a diuretic (Graham & Pettinger 1979) when its full effect in reducing total cholesterol is preserved. Its use in this way, rather than in combination with a beta-blocker, should become more widespread as appreciation of the importance of cholesterol control increases. Fixed combinations would be difficult because there is such wide variation in effective dosage, ranging from 2 to 20 mg/day.

CALCIUM BLOCKERS

Only one calcium channel blocker, nifedipine, has come into general use as an antihypertensive in Britain. Though verapamil has been available for much longer, and has recently been promoted as an antihypertensive drug, its complex effects on heart muscle and the heart's conducting system make it essentially a tool for cardiologists, not GPs.

Nifedipine relaxes smooth muscle in the arterial and arteriolar walls in hypertensives, reducing peripheral resistance without a compensatory increase in heart output, so that blood pressure falls. Angina is usually controlled by reducing heart workload and coronary spasm, and nifedipine is a useful combination with, or alternative to, beta-blockers for this purpose. There is usually some increase in heart rate at first, but this generally disappears after a few weeks. The standard preparation often causes headaches, palpitation and flushing, and must be given three or four times a day, so it is probably best always to use the slow-release preparation which can be given twice a day and is much less likely to cause these side-effects. It may cause menorrhagia (Rodger & Torrance 1983). There is wide variability in individual response, and doses up to 60 mg/day may be needed.

Apart from flushing and headache in about 5% of patients with the standard preparation (less with the slow-release form) there seem to be few short-term side-effects. It is too soon as yet to know much about long-term effects, positive or negative, though there is a reduction in plasma potassium which could be worrying if combined with the effect of most diuretics. If diuretics are used with nifedipine, it is probably best to choose a potassium-sparing sort such as amiloride (Murphy et al 1983). There is hope that nifedipine may have a useful inhibiting effect on platelet aggregation. So far as I know there is no information about long-term effects on blood cholesterol.

Nifedipine seems to have few contraindications. It should not be used in combination with beta-blockers in the presence of poor left ventricular function, shown by enlargement of the heart or frank heart failure. In a few patients it may, paradoxically, precipitate rather than relieve angina.

ANGIOTENSIN CONVERTING ENZYME INHIBITORS

ACE inhibitors arrived with captopril in 1981, which was at first used in unnecessarily high doses (around 300 mg/day) which led to frequent side-effects, mainly proteinuria, reduction in white blood cells and taste disturbances. In the 50–100 mg daily dosage used now, these side-effects are rare. Enalapril was introduced in 1984, with even fewer apparent side-effects and once-daily dosage.

Both are usually effective in reducing blood pressure, and their effect is greatly increased by combination with a diuretic and/or moderate reduction of sodium intake to around 100 mmol/day. Be careful not to use a potassium-sparing diuretic like amiloride, triamterene or spironolactone, which, together with an ACE inhibitor may cause a dangerous rise in blood potassium. Rebound hypertension has not been reported after withdrawal of either drug.

Enalapril generally causes fewer side-effects in day-to-day use than alternative antihypertensive drugs, but it is early days yet, and patients who have changed from an old to a new antihypertensive drug usually report benefits which are not felt by newly diagnosed hypertensives starting treatment for the first time. An important and credible interpretation of the unexpected results of the MRC mild hypertension trial, which showed a big reduction in stroke deaths with diuretics but not with propranolol, has been presented by Brown and Brown (1986). They suggest that, because regulation of blood pressure in small brain arteries depends on angiotensin II, ACE inhibitors may actually increase the risk of intracerebral haemorrhage, despite the reduction in the brachial artery pressure which we normally measure. Until we have more evidence on this, it seems unwise to adopt ACE inhibitors as first or second line drugs.

Otherwise, there seem to be three main problems with ACE inhibitors; early hypotension, precipitation of renal failure, and rapid sodium depletion and collapse in the event of diarrhoea form an intercurrent illness.

Early hypotension with faintness tends to occur in patients who are already sodium-depleted by diet, diuretics or both, and is more likely with captopril than enalapril. Neither drug should ever be started simultaneously with a diuretic, and if a diuretic already in use cannot be withdrawn, the ACE inhibitor should be introduced cautiously, with advice to take a long salty drink if faintness occurs.

Patients on the edge of renal failure depend on circulating angiotension to maintain arterial flow through the kidney. An ACE inhibitor may therefore precipitate kidney failure, and patients started on these drugs should have a repeat measurement of urea and creatinine about 2 weeks after they start, to compare with the pretreatment baseline measurement.

The last possibility, collapse with water and sodium depletion with what might otherwise be a minor and self-limiting diarrhoea, seems to me the most likely cause of serious iatrogenic illness once these drugs begin to be used on a mass scale, as no doubt they soon will be. Patients started on ACE inhibitors should be told that these drugs work by impeding the normal mechanism for correcting salt and water depletion in diarrhoea, and that in the event of such an intercurrent illness, increased intake of fluids containing added salt at a rate of one level teaspoonful to each litre is essential. The possibilities of unexpected acute illness on exotic *costas* can be imagined.

Of the two ACE inhibitors now available, enalapril seems the obvious clinical choice, though it is even more expensive.

REFERENCES

Bai T R, Webb D, Hamilton M et al 1982 Treatment of hypertension with beta-adrenoreceptor blocking drugs. Journal of the Royal College of Physicians of London 16:239

Berglund G, Andersson O 1981 Beta-blockers or diuretics in hypertension? A six year follow-up of blood pressure and metabolic side-effects. Lancet i:744

Bing R F, Russell G I, Thurston H et al 1980 Hydralazine in hypertension: is there a safe dose? British Medical Journal 280:353

Bogaert M G, Clement D L 1983 Lack of influence of propranolol and metoprolol on walking distance in patients with chronic intermittent claudication. European Heart Journal 4:203

Breckenridge A 1983 Which beta blocker? British Medical Journal 286:1085

Brown M J, Brown J 1986 Does angiotensin II protect against strokes? Lancet ii:427

Cameron H A, Ramsay L E 1983 Which beta-blocker? British Medical Journal 286:1439.

Carstairs K, Worlledges, Dollery C T et al 1966 Methyldopa and haemolytic anaemia. Lancet ii:201

Coope J R 1983 Reduction of ventricular ectopic beats in older subjects on atenolol: relation to serum potassium levels. Journal of Hypertension 1:342

de Swiet M 1985 Antihypertensive drugs in pregnancy. British Medical Journal 291:365

Donovan M A, Heagerty A M, Patel L et al 1981 Cimetidine and bioavailability of propranolol. Lancet i:164

Fairley K F, Birch D F, Haines I 1983 Abnormal urinary sediment in patients on triamterene. Lancet i:421

Fidler J, Smith V, Fayers P et al 1983 Randomised controlled comparative study of methyldopa and oxprenolol in treatment of hypertension in pregnancy. British Medical Journal 286:1927

Goldberg A D, Raftery E B, Wilkinson P 1977 Blood pressure and heart rate and withdrawal of antihypertensive drugs. British Medical Journal i:1243

Graham R M, Pettinger W A 1979 Prazosin. New England Journal of Medicine 300:232

Harth M 1968 L E cells and positive direct Coomb's test induced by methyldopa. Canadian Medical Association Journal 99:227

Hoyumpa A M, Connell A M 1973 Methyldopa hepatitis. American Journal of Digestive Diseases 18:213

Jarrett R J 1983 Thiazide diuretics and glucose tolerance. Lancet i:72

Johnson B F, Saunders R, Hickler R et al 1986 The effects of thiazide diuretics upon plasma lipoproteins. Journal of Hypertension 4:235

Kirch W, Kohler H, Spahn H et al 1981 Interaction of cimetidine with metoprolol, propranolol, or atenolol. Lancet ii:531

Leren P, Foss P O, Helgeland A et al 1980 Effect of propranolol and prazosin on blood lipids; the Oslo study. Lancet ii:4

McMahon F G 1978 Management of essential hypertension. Futura Publishing, New York. Seven studies comparing side-effects of reserpine with other antihypertensive drugs are reviewed on p 344

McMahon F G, Ryan J R, Akdamal K et al 1982 Upper gastrointestinal lesions after potassium chloride supplements: a controlled clinical trial. Lancet ii:1059

Mansilla-Tinoco R, Harland S J, Ryan P J et al 1982 Hydralazine, antinuclear antibodies, and the lupus syndrome. British Medical Journal 284:936

Medical Research Council Working Party on mild to moderate hypertension 1981 Adverse reactions to bendrofluazide and propranolol for the treatment of mild hypertension. Lancet ii:539

Medical Research Council Working Party 1985 MRC trial of mild hypertension: principal results. British Medical Journal 291:97

Morgan D B, Davidson C 1980 Hypokalaemia and diuretics: an analysis of publications. British Medical Journal ii:905

Murphy M B, Lewis P J, Kohner E et al 1982 Glucose intolerance in hypertensive patients treated with diuretics: a fourteen-year follow-up. Lancet ii:1293

Murphy M B, Scriven A J I, Dollery C T 1983 Role of nifedipine in treatment of hypertension. British Medical Journal 287:257

Opie L H 1984 Drugs and the heart four years on. Lancet i:496

Ounsted M, Moar V, Redman C W G et al 1980 Infant growth and development following treatment of maternal hypertension. Lancet 1980; i:705.

Pitts N E 1974 The clinical evaluation of prazosin hydrochloride. In: Cotton D W K (ed) Prazosin: evaluation of a new antihypertensive agent. Excerpta Medica, Amsterdam, p 149

Pryor J P, Castle W M 1982 Peyronie's disease associated with chronic degenerative arterial disease and not with beta-adrenoceptor blocking agents. Lancet i:917

Pryor J P, Castle W M, Dukes D C et al 1983 Do beta-adrenoceptor blocking drugs cause retroperitoneal fibrosis? British Medical Journal 287:639

Ramsay L E 1981 The use of methyldopa in the elderly. Journal of the Royal College of Physicians of London 15:239

Reid J L, Wing L M H, Dargie H J et al 1977 Clonidine withdrawal in hypertension: changes in blood pressure and plasma and urinary noradrenaline. Lancet i:1171

Rodger J C, Torrance T C 1983 Can nifedipine provoke menorrhagia? Lancet ii:460

Sandor F F, Pickens P T, Crallan J 1982 Variations of plasma potassium concentrations during long-term treatment of hypertension with diuretics without potassium supplements. British Medical Journal 284:711

Sataline L, Lowell D 1976 Methyldopa toxicity. Gastroenterology 70:149

Thomas J P, Thomson W H 1983 Comparison of thiazides and amiloride in treatment of moderate hypertension. British Medical Journal 286:2015

Veterans Administration Co-operative Group on antihypertensive agents 1977 Propranolol in the treatment of essential hypertension. Journal of the American Medical Association 237:2303

Veterans Administration Co-operative Group on antihypertensive agents 1982a Low dose versus standard dose of reserpine: a randomised, double-blind, multiclinic trial in patients taking chlorthalidone. Journal of the American Medical Association 248:2471

Veterans Administration Co-operative Study Group on antihypertensive agents 1982b Comparison of propranolol and hydrochlorothiazide for the initial treatment of hypertension. I. Results of short-term titration with emphasis on racial differences. Journal of the American Medical Association 248:1996

18

Refractory and complicated cases

Audit of the care of any large number of hypertensives generally shows about 20% well above target pressure. Two medical errors and seven groups of patients account for nearly all these cases.

The two medical errors are:

1. Not to titrate each drug to a point where side-effects or the risk of them preclude higher dosage, and to assume that because a drug appears to be ineffective on its own, it will also be ineffective in combination (Mackay 1983)

2. Inadvertent prescription of drugs which either raise blood pressure or oppose the action of antihypertensive medication. The commonest of these are NSAIDs such as indomethacin. Indomethacin almost completely nullifies the hypotensive effect of propranolol and thiazide diuretics (Watkins et al 1980). Neither beta-blockers nor thiazides should be used for hypertension in patients dependent on these drugs for control of inflammatory joint disease. Use of NSAIDs for non-inflammatory joint pain is both common and ineffective. Other possibilities are oral contraceptives, para-sympathomimetic amines used as nasal vasoconstrictors or appetite suppressants, and carbenoxolone. All antidepressant drugs oppose the action of antihypertensive drugs to some extent, and depressive illness is itself a cause of hypertension. Phenothiazine drugs used for psychotic illness can interact with methyldopa to cause a paradoxical rise in blood pressure (Westervelt & Atuk 1974).

The seven groups of patients are:

1. Patients who persistently fail to take their drugs. Absence of bradycardia in patients on beta-blockers or reserpine suggests non-compliance. About half of all patients in most published series show major problems of non-compliance 3 months after starting medication. If readings are above target pressure, ask first whether

the last dose has been taken yet. Repeated admission that a recent dose has been omitted often indicates a more general pattern of non-compliance which some patients find difficult to admit. The problems of compliance are discussed in Chapter 13.

2. Patients drinking large amounts of alcohol, above approximate thresholds of 80 g/day in men or 40 g/day in women (80 g alcohol = 4 pints of beer, 8 glasses of wine, or 4 double measures of spirits). This is in my experience the commonest cause of refractory hypertension. Useful clues are raised mean corpuscular volume (which can sometimes be tracked back for years on previous full blood count reports), raised gamma GT transferase, smell of alcohol, flushed face and palms, and morning nausea or vomiting, particularly after weekends.

3. Patients exposed to an intractable background of stress at home or at work. This may operate directly, as well as by causing poor compliance and alcohol dependence.

4. Patients who seem to be intolerant of nearly all antihypertensive drugs. If this seems to be happening, it is worth trying the effect of placebo (e.g. ascorbic acid 50 mg twice a day) to see if this also causes side-effects; if so, the finding should be discussed with the patient, who may then be able to recognise anxiety as the real cause of the symptoms.

5. Patients in whom antihypertensive drugs are initially effective, but seem later to become ineffective. All commonly used antihypertensive drugs except diuretics and beta-blockers may induce sodium and water retention, with expansion of plasma volume and a rise in blood pressure. Addition of a diuretic, increased dosage of a diuretic already in use, or a change to one of greater potency will usually restore control. Secondary renal artery stenosis can simulate this.

6. Patients with unrecognised secondary hypertension. Rapid escalation of previously well controlled pressure may signify acquired renal artery stenosis, or some other cause of renal damage. Rare causes of secondary hypertension such as aldosterone-secreting tumours and phaeochromocytoma are more likely to be detected because of anomalous non-response to normally adequate antihypertensive treatment than by investigations before treatment begins.

7. Patients who are resistant to all the drugs normally used. These are candidates for ACE inhibitors plus a diuretic. At one time they would have been treated, in men at least, with minoxidil.

Uncontrolled severe hypertension is a high risk, and if you cannot control diastolic pressures below 100 mmHg after 3 months in patients with initial diastolic pressures of 115 mmHg or more, the patients should be referred to a cardiologist with a serious interest in hypertension, and be prepared to operate some system of shared care (Swales 1984). Referral to a cardiologist who applies only a standard set of elementary investigations which you should already have done yourself, and then delegates indefinite follow-up to a succession of junior staff, is no service to the patient. Everyone with long experience of antihypertensive treatment agrees that patients who are initially difficult to control often become easily controlled after a few years, sometimes with simple drug regimens which were originally ineffective. This may be because of improved compliance, or it may be that partial control for a few years changes the body's response to treatment. Persistence pays off in the end; half a loaf is not only better than no bread, but sometimes preferable to entering the pipeline of high technology investigation and experimental treatment.

MANAGEMENT OF HYPERTENSION WITH CONCURRENT DIABETES

In October 1985 I had 28 adult diabetics in a population of 1200 people aged 20 and over — roughly 2% of that population — which is about the expected number for full ascertainment. Twelve of these were on concurrent antihypertensive treatment, with a group mean pretreatment pressure of 203/114 mmHg (mean of three readings, phase V). There is a positive association between blood pressure and glucose intolerance, as one would expect since obesity is a causal factor for both, so in any group of hypertensives there will be more diabetes than in the general population. More important still, the control of high blood pressure and of other coronary and stroke risk factors is much more important in diabetics than in the general population. Diabetics die not of diabetes but of its vascular complications: chiefly early coronary disease, stroke, peripheral arterial disease, and renal failure. Blood pressure control is therefore more important in diabetics, and probably more effective, and there is a good case (though so far as I know no controlled evidence) for treatment in diabetics from a mean diastolic threshold of 90 mmHg (phase V).

Because all diuretics seem to impair glucose tolerance in about 20% of patients after 2 or 3 years (Murphy et al 1982), they should be avoided as a first-line treatment in diabetics, in the very obese, and in patients with a history of diabetes in first degree relatives. It is not possible altogether to avoid their use in these groups, and when they are used this risk should be borne in mind, and dosage kept to a minimum. In insulin-dependent diabetics, diuretics can precipitate ketoacidosis and should be used cautiously if at all, though thiazides are safer than frusemide in this respect. For maturity-onset diabetics, the diabetogenic effect of diuretics is not large and many people gain far more than they are likely to lose by their use.

There is no evidence that prolonged treatment with beta-blockers impairs glucose tolerance (Vedin et al 1975), but the upward shift in total cholesterol is more dangerous for diabetics than other hypertensives and beta-blockers should be avoided if possible. They have no effect on blood glucose control in non-insulin-dependent diabetes (Wright et al 1979), but may mask the warning symptoms of hypoglycaemia in brittle diabetics.

Nifedipine, prazosin and ACE inhibitors seem to be the best drugs to choose from for diabetics, but diuretics will be necessary for many of them.

MANAGEMENT OF HYPERTENSION WITH CONCURRENT AIRWAYS OBSTRUCTION

In Glyncorrwg in October 1985, of 132 hypertensives identified by screening and currently being followed up, 46 (35%) had substantial airways obstruction (peak expiratory flow rate <300 l/min, and/or increasing by 20% or more after inhaled salbutamol). The proportion was somewhat higher than in the population as a whole (22%). Clearly substantial airways obstruction is a common complicating factor in the treatment of hypertension.

Continued smoking is an urgent problem both for hypertensives and for those with airways obstruction, and when both of these are combined the control of smoking should take priority over all other measures. Beta-blockers are contraindicated absolutely for patients with reversible airways obstruction; a daily dose as low as 40 mg can cause death in young asthmatics, whose PEFR in the small hours may be far lower than anything recorded during the day. If this emergency does nevertheless occur, the best immediate treatment is an intravenous injection of salbutamol or isoprenaline together with intravenous glucagon (Harries 1981). Where airways obstruction is fixed, beta-blockers may safely be used, but only with caution and after a formal test of airways responsiveness in the surgery. If PEFR does not increase by 15% or more 20 minutes after inhaling 400 μg salbutamol, a cardioselective beta-blocker such as atenolol or metoprolol can be used cautiously, if PEFR is monitored regularly at follow-up. At very low PEFR, below 120 l/min or so, it is unwise to use beta-blockers of any kind, even if obstruction is not reversible.

MANAGEMENT OF HYPERTENSION WITH CONCURRENT RENAL FAILURE

Though primary hypertension short of the malignant phase is almost never a direct cause of renal failure, virtually all kinds of acute or chronic renal damage tend to raise blood pressure, which in turn accelerates the decline of renal function. Assiduous control of blood pressure is the most important preventive measure that can be taken for patients in the early stages of renal failure, and is the only way to slow progression of renal damage in diabetics.

Use of drugs in end-stage renal failure, in which dialysis, transplant or terminal illness are imminent, is outside the scope of this book. All GPs have to assist in management of such patients, but decisions on medication will be taken by specialists. The following remarks apply to early renal failure, when the aim is to conserve whatever renal function is left, and avoid iatrogenic illness from clumsy use of drugs. Many such patients will already be beginning to restrict protein and dietary sodium, and should be known to the nearest dialysis/transplant unit so that contingency plans can be made for future management.

It is essential to keep medication as simple as possible. No drugs should be used that are not absolutely necessary, and a high priority should be given to control of blood pressure.

Thiazide diuretics are ineffective in patients with less than 20% renal function (Reubi & Cottier 1961) measured by creatinine clearance, and can precipitate acute renal failure. Spironolactone and other potassium-sparing diuretics should not be used because of the risk of exacerbating hyperkalaemia. Early symptomless renal failure is common in the elderly, and antihypertensive treatment should not be started without initial measurement of urea and creatinine. Frusemide is a safe alternative diuretic.

Methyldopa can be used in renal failure in much reduced dosage, but it is rarely wise to use such a toxic drug. Beta-blockers, prazosin and nifedipine can be used safely, though it is always wise to titrate from a low dose, with changes at intervals of not less than 2 days.

ACE inhibitors are cleared through the kidney, and are therefore cumulative in renal failure. They can also reduce perfusion through the renal parenchyma, leading to a decline in renal function despite good control of blood pressure. Initial dosage should be very small, diuretics should only be added later, and renal function should be monitored.

REFERENCES

Harries A D 1981 Beta-blockade in asthma. British Medical Journal 282:1321

Mackay A Management of intractable hypertension. Journal of the Royal Society of Medicine 76:537

Murphy M B, Lewis P J, Kohner E et al 1982 Glucose intolerance in hypertensive patients treated with diuretics: a fourteen-year follow-up. Lancet ii:1293

Reubi F C, Cottier P T 1961 Effect of reduced glomerular filtration rate on responsiveness to chlorothiazide and mercurial diuretics. Circulation 23:200

Swales J D 1984 Treating severe hypertension. Journal of the Royal College of Physicians of London 18:46

Vedin A, Wilhelmsson C, Bjorntorp P 1975 Induction of diabetes and oral glucose tolerance tests during and after chronic beta-blockade. Acta Medica Scandinavica (suppl 575):37

Watkins J, Abbott E C, Hensby C N et al 1980 Attenuation of hypotensive effect of propranolol and thiazide diuretics by indomethacin. British Medical Journal 281:702

Westervelt F B, Atuk N O 1974 Methyldopa-induced hypertension. Journal of the American Medical Association 227:557

Wright A D, Barber S G, Kendall M J et al 1979 Beta-adrenoceptor-blocking drugs and blood sugar control in diabetes mellitus. British Medical Journal i:159

19

Hypertension in childhood and youth

This chapter deals with three important themes: how not to miss the once-in-a-lifetime case of immediately serious hypertension in childhood, what we should do about the possible origins of adult hypertension in childhood, and what we should do about the by no means rare cases of hypertension between 20 and 40 years of age. As before, we are discussing detection and management in general practice; availability of skilled back-up by hospital-based specialists is assumed.

MEASUREMENT OF BLOOD PRESSURE IN CHILDHOOD

The considerable difficulties of guaranteeing accurate and representative measurement of arterial pressure in adults are vastly greater in childhood. A full range of child-size cuffs is essential, which means at least three different sizes to cover the age range 5–15. Table 19.1 shows the cuff sizes proposed by a WHO expert committee (1978). Under 4 years of age a Doppler ultrasound recorder with earphones and an acoustic head is essential to pick up a systolic signal, and diastolic pressure cannot be reliably measured at all. Measurement of blood pressure under 5 years of age is a research exercise requiring special training and experience, and though there is every reason why GPs interested in longitudinal population studies should undertake this work, it has no real connection with current clinical practice. In Glyncorrwg our research team recorded systolic pressures monthly in a cohort of infants and we have followed them annually since 1977. We have confirmed what everyone else working in this field already knows: blood pressure in infancy and childhood is far more variable than in adults, so that many more readings have to be taken to characterise an individual as ranking high or low in a population distribution; artefacts related mainly to cuff size and method of picking up the systolic signal can introduce huge measurement

Table 19.1 Appropriate cuff sizes for various applications proposed by a WHO expert committee

Subject	Bladder width (cm)	Bladder length (cm)
Newborns	2.5–4.0	5.0–10.0
Infants	6.0–8.0	12.0–13.5
Children	9.0–10.0	17.0–22.5

Table 19.2 Blood pressure recordings in three primary schoolchildren

Mean school reading (mmHg)	Follow-up reading (mmHg)
158/126	108/56
137/105	108/54
154/94	90/56

errors, and children examined in schools are subject to very large effects from apprehension which may not be obvious. For example, I examined 15 11-year-old children in the last school clinic we held, and three had diastolic pressures over 90 mmHg confirmed by two replicate readings. We followed them up at the health centre a week later with the results which are given in Table 19.2.

A further problem which intrudes on clinical measurements of blood pressure in later childhood is that normal blood pressure relates to stature as well as to age. Children in any given age band show a wider dispersion of stature (weight for height; body mass index is not an appropriate measure for children) than adults, because they vary so much in development. Around the time of the adolescent growth spurt, usually between the ages of 12 and 17, children are almost members of different species, and ranking for blood pressure is absurd unless development is taken into account as well as stature.

IMMEDIATELY SERIOUS HYPERTENSION IN CHILDHOOD

A sustained blood pressure of say 145/95 mmHg in a child of 12 is unusual enough to require careful follow-up and some elementary investigations, but it is not a medical emergency. Unless it is found to rise higher over the next few days or weeks, it is not in the category considered here.

Clinical hypertension in childhood is secondary hypertension; primary ('essential') hypertension probably already exists, but it is not a clinical problem. Of children with a diastolic pressure >120 mmHg, 95% have an identifiable cause of secondary hypertension (Still & Cottorn 1967). Secondary hypertension in childhood is overwhelmingly renal, from acute glomerulonephritis, from renin-secreting tumours, from renal malformations already approaching end-stage renal failure, occasionally from nephroblastoma (Wilms tumour), though this presents as a mass in the flank rather than as raised blood pressure alone. Coarctation of the aorta usually presents during the first year of life, but children who survive to the second year without symptoms generally seem healthy, and tend to be picked up from investigation of a systolic murmur. Blood pressure is not necessarily very high; it is the difference between arm and leg pressures which is important.

Headache is a common symptom in childhood, and is usually migrainous, often accompanied or for several years preceded by spells of abdominal pain. Pallor during the attack is usual, and initial visual spectra are frequently present if asked for, though for some unaccountable reason children hardly ever describe these on their own initiative. Even with a classical history of migraine, all children complaining of headache should have a careful examination of both optic fundi (nearly always easy with the large pupils of childhood), and all of them should have their blood pressure measured.

Though severe hypertension in childhood is rare, when it does occur it seems usually to be overlooked until organ damage is already advanced, and often irreversible. Three children aged 11–12 admitted to the Hospital for Sick Children at Great Ormond Street with neurovascular damage were found to have previously unrecorded blood pressures of 270/180, 280/190 and 190/110 mmHg 10 weeks, 9 months and 4 years respectively after their first presentation with morning headache (Hulse et al 1979). Two became permanently blind and one was left with permanent gross visual field defects, and one became paraplegic. All had renal hypertension.

POSSIBLE ORIGINS OF ADULT HYPERTENSION IN CHILDHOOD

It is perhaps not surprising that high ranking for blood pressure in infancy tends to be associated with high ranking for blood pressure years and decades later, the phenomenon known as 'tracking'. It should not be surprising, because most other characteristics also show some degree of tracking: weight for height, skinfold thickness, airways reactivity, reading proficiency, and the tendency to pick one's nose. Blood pressure increases with age throughout childhood, and is also closely associated with growth (represented by height), obesity (represented by weight for height and by skinfold thickness), and development (represented by Tanner sexual development staging (Tanner 1962)). Since rankings for height and obesity do not vary randomly between periodic measurements in a cohort (and we would be very surprised if they did), why should we not expect blood pressure to behave in this way? In fact, stability of ranking for blood pressure in a cohort can be represented in two ways; as a tendency for successive rankings to resemble one another ('tracking'), and as a tendency for successive rankings to differ ('untracking'?). Both tendencies are important, and both are obscured by the true variability of blood pressure around its mean value, and by measurement difficulties, particularly in young children.

All this must be said, because though the idea that adult hypertension begins in childhood is strategically important and biologically plausible, it does not have to be true. There are other nodal points in development, notably adolescence and the early reproductive years, which are no less likely as starting points for the development of hypertension. Almost the only thing we can be sure of is that hypertension does not begin in the age-group in which it is usually recognised, from 40–65.

Longitudinal studies of blood pressure and other risk factors for coronary disease have been made in cohorts of children in Britain (Darby & Fearn 1979; de Swiet et al 1980), in the Netherlands following early initiatives by de Haas (van der Haar & Kromhout 1978), and in the USA in Boston (Kass et al 1977) and in the Bogalusa study in Louisiana (Berenson et al 1980), a sort of childhood Framingham. Studies from all non-socialist countries have been reviewed by Labarthe (1983). Another multicentre longitudinal study of 19 000 children born in 1964 began in Budapest, Moscow, Kaunas (Lithuania), East Berlin, Havana, and Ulan Bator (Mongolia) in 1975 (Török 1979).

Studies in Dunedin, New Zealand (Simpson et al 1981) are of particular interest because they measured socioeconomic correlates of blood pressure at birth, at 3 years of age, and at 7 in a cohort of more than 1000 children. No associations were found with socioeconomic status, maternal intelligence, maternal or paternal education, breast-feeding, or language development or observed behaviour in the child. Several US studies have shown that the divergence between blacks and whites, which is a social as well as a racial difference, develops only after 7 or 8 years of age, and really spreads out during and after adolescence.

All studies show 'tracking' of blood pressure, increasing from correlation coefficients of 0.2–0.3 at 2 years to adult levels of 'tracking' at age 20. Zinner, for example, found that 65% of children with initial systolic pressures more than 1 standard deviation above the mean and 70% of children with initial systolic pressures more than 1 standard deviation below the mean remained in that rank 4 years later (Kass et al 1977).

The report of the United States Task Force on childhood hypertension (National Heart, Lung and Blood Institutes 1977) suggested that infants and children with sustained blood pressures above the 95th centile for age required a complete medical history and examination to determine the cause and to develop an appropriate follow-up programme. In US clinical practice, experts in this field now suggest that these children be considered

> legitimate candidates for sustained drug treatment. . . There is some preliminary information from studies with certain pharmacologic agents over the course of 5–7 years that major adverse effects due to these drugs are generally uncommon. That is not to say that adverse reactions do not occur in this population, but to indicate that the incidence and effects noted do not differ significantly from those observed in adults (Kotchen & Kotchen 1981).

That such a proposal can be seriously discussed in our present state of ignorance seems extraordinary; nothing is more dangerous than doctors with potent weapons, an available target, a rational strategy, lacking only the empirical evidence of randomised trials which are the only conceivable justification for opening fire. A 20-year follow-up of young Czechs aged 14–26 with arterial pressures at or over 170/100 mmHg and not treated showed that only 17% had progressed to higher pressures, none had retinopathy, and one-third had diastolic pressures <90 mmHg (Widimsky & Jandova 1980).

The US Task Force report has stimulated detection programmes of some kind in the schools medical service in many parts of Britain, presumably leading to the referral of many children to district hospital paediatricians for investigation and assessment. A few of these will have clinical hypertension (nearly all of it secondary) which we know how to manage with ultimate benefit to the patient. Nearly all the 'cases' found will be children with more or less stable primary hypertension, and the truth is that we simply do not have the evidence to justify any programme of long-term medication for any of these children. Weight reduction, and less certainly some reduction in dietary sodium, are the only interventions likely to help these children, and this should be organised on a group rather than an individual basis, because children will only change their behaviour if they have group support. To tell these children and their parents that they are at high risk would, on present evidence, be untrue and irresponsible, but there is no need for this, since control of obesity is an acceptable target in its own right.

Figure 19.1 shows the centile distribution for boys and girls in the first year of life (from the Brompton study (de Swiet et al 1980)), and for boys only from the age of 1+ to 18 from centres in Miami, Muscatine and Rochester USA. This is only a very rough guide, because it does not allow for differences in stature and development, and because even with the greatest care, different

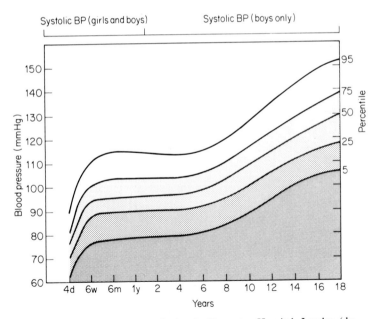

Fig. 19.1 Research up to 12 months by the Brompton Hospital, London (de Swiet et al 1980); 18 months onwards from centres in Miami, Muscatine and Rochester, USA (Berenson et al 1981).

research programmes on similar populations show as much as 10 mmHg difference between the same centile lines for systolic and diastolic pressures (Berenson et al 1981).

CAN ADULT HYPERTENSION BE PREVENTED BY CONTROL OF OBESITY IN CHILDHOOD?

All cross-sectional studies show an association between obesity and blood pressure in childhood. The effect of weight is independent of age and height (Voors & Berenson 1981). White US children in the upper third of the distribution of blood pressure are about 15 kg heavier than those in the bottom third, and 1 hour after an oral glucose load their blood glucose is about 15 mg/dl higher; after controlling for weight, there is still an independent association of blood pressure with blood glucose, particularly in children with evidence of peripheral insulin resistance. These associations seem to be absent in black children.

Several controlled intervention studies are under way in different parts of the world to test the hypothesis that control of obesity in childhood may prevent later onset of hypertension. The short-term results so far available suggest that blood pressure and blood cholesterol do fall in the intervention groups, and it is reasonable to suppose that this can eventually lead to a substantial fall in coronary and stroke risk. Because both high blood pressure and obesity are strongly inherited, we cannot assume that obesity control will necessarily have the full effect we hope for, but it is certainly reasonable to act now on the assumption that it will.

CAN ADULT HYPERTENSION BE PREVENTED BY CONTROL OF DIETARY SODIUM IN CHILDHOOD?

Rigorously designed and carefully performed studies in young teenage children have failed to show any significant association between urinary sodium output (the only way to measure intake) and blood pressure (Cooper et al 1983). A small positive association has been shown in infants (Hofman et al 1983). Offspring of parents in the top and bottom thirds of the distribution of blood pressure both show no change in blood pressure in response to reductions in sodium intake of 50% or more over 4 weeks (Watt et al 1985), nor do they show any difference in avidity for sodium (Watt et al 1983). Nevertheless, average American and west European diets contain far more sodium than is necessary, and big reductions are possible if undertaken slowly. Experimental evidence that this will reduce blood pressure, or prevent later hypertension, is as yet unconvincing. It is still likely, despite the weakness of experimental evidence so far available, that excess dietary sodium sustained over years rather than weeks does interact with genetic factors as the principal cause of primary hypertension. If this is so, it is also likely that this effect occurs mainly in childhood, and is reversible at that time by reduction in sodium load.

Where such a reduction can be made easily, without obstructing other measures for which there is better experimental support (reduction in dietary fat, for example), it should certainly be done. Contrary to most of our assumptions, snack foods and added table salt contribute little to teenage sodium intake. Table 19.3 shows the percentage distribution of various sources of dietary sodium in the diet of 200 US high school students aged 15–17, with an average daily sodium intake of 170 mmol for boys and 110 mmol for girls (Ellison et al 1986). This reflects US eating patterns, in which bottled sauces largely replace added table salt, but it emphasises usefully the large contribution from bread and other cereal products. As these form a large part of most fibre-rich diets, there is potential conflict between the aims of fat reduction and sodium reduction.

Table 19.3 Percentage distribution of various sources of sodium in adolescent diets in the USA

Food group	% Na intake
Cereals	30
Meat, fish, eggs	21
Sauces, dressings, etc.	19
Fruit, vegetables	16
Snack foods	6
Added table salt	<1

The most important contribution to reduced sodium load in childhood would be a return to free school meals with a planned menu adapted both to teenage tastes and to health needs.

CONCLUSION ON BLOOD PRESSURE IN CHILDHOOD

GPs, school doctors and community paediatricians should none of us ignore arterial pressure in childhood, but we should learn to observe before we intervene, except for the occasional case of symptomatic severe hypertension. Action to control childhood obesity could probably best be developed by group work as a part of the school medical service. Reductions in sodium load by about 20% would not be difficult, by modifying school meals and by pressure on the manufacturers of prepared foods, but this should not be allowed to conflict with better validated changes in diet, particularly reductions in dietary fat.

MANAGEMENT OF HYPERTENSION IN YOUTH

This is a more serious and immediate clinical problem for most GPs than childhood hypertension, because there is a lot of it about, and very little evidence on which to base a responsible policy. From the complete screen for hypertension in Glyncorrwg in 1968 and in the following 18 years, from a total population of 2000 we have had 29 with systolic pressures at or over 160 mmHg, or diastolic pressures at or over 100 mmHg, on the mean of three consecutive readings. All readings were with a random zero sphygmomanometer and outsize cuffs where appropriate. Only one of these had a classical cause of secondary hypertension (obstructive uropathy). Some characteristics of the 28 patients who might have been ascribed to 'essential hypertension' are shown in Table 19.4.

Table 19.4 Some characteristics of 28 young 'primary' hypertensives in Glyncorrwg, 1969–1986

	Men (n = 16)	Women (n = 11)
Mean age at diagnosis	34.4	32.1
Range	31–39	18–39
Mean blood pressure at diagnosis	166.8/107.6	171.5/109.2
Range	150–202/102–130	144–220/91–155
BMI > 30	5	2
BMI < 25	3	7
Alcohol problem	9 (7 confirmed)	1 + 2 doubtful

Striking differences between men and women are concealed within the fairly small difference in incidence (16 men and 12 women from male and female populations of almost identical size). Although this was not understood at the time, alcohol was clearly a principal or important contributory cause in more than half the men, and all but three of them were overweight. One of these men moved away and died of perforated diverticulitis soon after the screening programme started, but of the other 14 all but three have had to remain on antihypertensive medication ever since. One of the three exceptions attained normal pressures when his alcohol intake (average 10 pints of beer daily) was drastically reduced, and has never needed medication. Another was able to stop medication after more than 10 years of good control, without any serious rise in pressure. The third is still under review before reaching a decision about treatment.

Only one woman had a serious alcohol problem, and her blood pressure quickly became normal whenever her drinking was reduced. In two others alcohol was unlikely but not excluded. Hypertension was related to oral contraception in over half the women, and in four of these blood pressure became normal soon after the pill was stopped. Three others have had to continue medication. Two women had a very serious weight problem (BMI 39.1 and 42.0).

Good blood pressure data were available on parents and/or siblings for 8 of the men and 6 of the women. Seven out of 8 men and 5 out of 6 women had one or both parents and/or a sibling with hypertension above our threshold for treatment.

MOST OF THE CAUSES OF HYPERTENSION IN YOUTH ARE KNOWN

Though the numbers are small, they are complete, and drawn from a defined population, so it seems reasonable to draw three important conclusions.

First of all, once blood pressures in the adult population are fully known, as they will be by applying policies of screening or case-finding over 5–10 years, accurate family data should be available for most patients. Nearly all the young hypertensives seem to come from subjects with high blood pressure in at least one first-degree relative, so the vulnerable group can be defined.

Secondly, within that vulnerable group, alcohol and obesity stand out as powerful accelerating factors. Both are reversible — not easily, but with less difficulty and with greater chances of success in young adults than in the middle-aged.

Finally, careful monitoring of oral contraception at 3 monthly intervals, as well as choice of lowest-dose combined preparations, should substantially reduce the incidence of hypertension in young women.

As yet we don't know all the causes of primary hypertension, but we already seem to know enough to make nonsense of the category. Not only is hypertension not essential, most of it is not even primary, but secondary to known and reversible causes acting against a fairly well defined (though certainly polygenic) genetic background.

A POLICY FOR YOUNG HYPERTENSIVES

Active search for young hypertensives, for men from age 20 when growth is complete, for women from the beginning of sexual activity, seems to be just as important as active search in middle age. An active call-up policy is justifiable for the offspring of hypertensive parents, or the younger siblings of known hypertensives.

Multiple readings and follow-up for at least 3 months before starting any medication are essential. People under 40 with mean pressures at or over 160/95 mmHg should be asked for a detailed account of their normal drinking habits through the week, checked with the spouse or other relative and by measurement of MCV and gamma GT. Height and weight should be measured, and plans made for nearest possible attainment of desirable body weight (BMI 25). Fasting lipids should be measured, both to assess coronary risk and give feedback on results after reducing dietary fat, and to assess triglyceride as a fairly consistent indicator of high alcohol intake. Cigarette smoking should be assessed and, if the patient agrees, a plan made for giving up, with priority for stopping smoking if there appears to be conflict with weight targets.

ANTIHYPERTENSIVE MEDICATION IN YOUTH

Though some harmful side-effects develop quickly within a month or two of starting antihypertensive medication, in general their risks are related to the number of years they are taken. A young man of 30 starting on a thiazide diuretic and a beta-blocker may receive them continuously for another 45 years or more, but the best evidence we have on long-term side-effects covers only 11 years for thiazides and 10 years propranolol. There are as yet no randomised controlled trials of the balance between risks and benefits for antihypertensive medication in this age group, and even if trials were to start now, there would have to be a lapse of at least 20 years before sufficient endpoints could accumulate to demonstrate any advantage for treatment. On the other hand, we have good reasons to believe that early control of blood pressure may be more effective than treatment in middle age, particularly in preventing atheroma and consequent coronary heart disease.

If we have to use drugs, which of them carry least risk and have fewest harmful side-effects for such very prolonged use? ACE inhibitors seem an obvious choice, but in my very limited experience they usually require concomitant diuretics to obtain good control at low dosage, and the long-term effects of diuretics are worrying. Prazosin is attractive because of its effect on blood cholesterol. The fatigue so often associated with beta-blockers, which is more frequent in younger and more physically active patients, and their cholesterol-raising effect, make them a poor choice in this age-group. Nifedipine seems to be well tolerated, but again it usually needs a thiazide. Whatever drug you choose, complete absence of symptomatic side-effects is essential if you are to expect long-term compliance. My guess is that most of these patients will in future be treated with enalapril, combined with the smallest possible dose of diuretic if necessary. This can only be justified if the diagnosis is made carefully, after repeated measurements during at least 2 or 3 months' observation before medication, and after serious attempts have been made to control obesity and alcohol intake.

REFERENCES

Berenson G S, McMahan C A, Voors A W et al 1980 Cardiovascular risk factors in children: the early natural history of atherosclerosis and essential hypertension. Oxford University Press, Oxford. This gives a full account of the Bogalusa study

Berenson G S, Voors A W, Webber L S 1981 Hypertension in the young: measurement and criteria. In: Onesti G, Kim K E (eds) Hypertension in the young and the old. Grune & Stratton, New York, p 3

Cooper R, Liu K, Trevisan M et al 1983 Urinary sodium excretion and blood pressure in children: absence of a reproducible association. Hypertension 5:135

Darby S C, Fearn T 1979 The Chatham blood pressure study: an application of Bayesian growth curve models to a longitudinal study of blood pressure in children. International Journal of Epidemiology 8:15

de Swiet M, Fayers P, Shinebourne E A 1980 Value of repeated blood pressure measurements in children — the Brompton study. British Medical Journal i:1567

Ellison R C, Capper A F, Witschi J C et al 1986 Sources of sodium intake in adolescents (abstract 174). CDV Epidemiology Newsletter (American Heart Association) no. 39, Winter

Hofman A, Hazebroek A, Valkenburg H A 1983 A randomised trial of sodium intake and blood pressure in newborn infants. Journal of the American Medical Association 250:370

Hulse J A, Taylor D S I, Dillon M J 1979 Blindness and paraplegia in severe childhood hypertension. Lancet ii:553

Kass E H, Rosner B, Zinner S H et al 1977 Studies on the origin of human hypertension. Postgraduate Medical Journal suppl 2:146

Kotchen J M, Kotchen T A 1981 Correlates of high blood pressure in adolescents. In Onesti G, Kim K E (eds) Hypertension in the young and the old. Grune & Stratton, New York, p 173

Labarthe D L 1983 Blood pressure studies in children throughout the world. In: Gross F, Strasser T (eds) Mild hypertension: recent advances. Raven Press, New York, p 85

National Heart, Lung and Blood Institutes 1977 Report of the Task Force on blood pressure control in children. Paediatrics 59 (suppl):797

Simpson A, Mortimer J G, Silva P A et al 1981 Correlates of blood pressure in a cohort of Dunedin seven-year-old children. In:Onesti G, Kim K E (eds) Hypertension in the young and the old. Grune & Stratton, New York, p 3

Still J L, Cottom D 1967 Severe hypertension in childhood. Archives of Disease in Childhood 43:34

Tanner J M 1962 Growth at adolescence. Blackwell, London

Torok E 1979 The beginnings of hypertension: studies in childhood and adolescence. In: Gross F, Strasser T (eds) Mild hypertension: natural history and management. Pitman Medical, London

van der Haar F, Kromhout D 1978 Food intake, nutritional anthropometry and blood chemical parameters in three selected Dutch school children populations. Veenman & Zonen BV, Wageningen, Netherlands

Voors A W, Berenson G S 1981 Search for the determinants of the early onset of essential hypertension. In: Onesti G, Kim K E (eds) Hypertension in the young and the old. Grune & Stratton, New York, p 43

Watt G C M, Foy C J W, Hart J T 1983 Comparison of blood pressure, sodium intake, and other variables in offspring with and without a family history of high blood pressure. Lancet i:1245

Watt G C M, Foy C J W, Hart J T et al 1985 Dietary sodium and arterial blood pressure: evidence against genetic susceptibility. British Medical Journal 291:1525

Widimsky J, Jandova R 1980 Long-term prognosis in juvenile hypertension: condition after 20 and 28 years (authors' translation). Casopis Lekaru Ceskych 119:1185

World Health Organization 1978 Arterial hypertension. WHO Technical Report series 628

20

Hypertension in the elderly

Slightly less than half the people treated for hypertension in Britain are aged 65 or over. High pressures and their lethal or disabling outcomes are much commoner in this age group, but so are some of the risks of medication, and so are deaths from other often more unpleasant causes. In the past few years we have at last got some good controlled trials of inception of antihypertensive medication in this age-group on which to base policies, but even more so than in younger patients, it is difficult to apply evidence derived from groups to decision making about individuals; old people vary enormously in their biological rather than chronological ages, in their accumulated burdens of diverse organ damage, and in their reasonable fears of other causes of death.

MEASUREMENT OF BLOOD PRESSURE IN OLD AGE

Despite some suggestions to the contrary (Spence et al 1978), indirect measurements of arterial pressure approximate more closely to intra-arterial pressures in the elderly than in younger subjects (Berliner et al 1961).

PROGRESSION OF BLOOD PRESSURE IN OLD AGE

In industrialised populations whose group mean pressures rise with age, diastolic pressure tends to fall in the age range 60 to 80, in men more than in women. This tendency is seen in both cohort and cross-sectional studies, so it is not just an effect of early deaths in men with high diastolic pressures (Spence et al 1978). Systolic pressure, however, continues to rise, though it flattens out in men from the age of about 70 onwards. From age 80, both systolic and diastolic pressures tend to fall in both sexes (Berliner et al 1961).

RISKS OF HIGH BLOOD PRESSURE IN THE ELDERLY

Up to about age 70, all prospective studies show a positive association between blood pressure and cardiovascular mortality, particularly from stroke. Contrary to traditional teaching, the association with systolic is even closer than with diastolic pressure (Kannel & Gordon 1978). The Framingham study showed no change in associated risk up to age 76, but in a British study of apparently healthy men aged 70-89, neither systolic nor diastolic pressure showed any association with survival (Anderson & Cowan 1976). Since then there has been other evidence from several countries (Hodkinson & Pomerance 1979; Evans et al 1980; Miall & Brennan 1981; Haavisto et al 1984) that from a threshold somewhere around 70 years, obviously depending more on biological than chronological age in individuals, neither systolic nor diastolic pressure has much prognostic significance.

The explanation for this seems to be that there is a J-curve in all-cause mortality in relation to both systolic and diastolic pressure, with raised mortality at very low as well as very high pressures (Miall & Brennan 1981; Coope et al 1985). Low pressures over the age of 70 are likely to be associated with previous myocardial infarction, atrial fibrillation, heart failure, cancer, or many other terminal illnesses associated with weight loss. This J-curve is more marked in women than men, reflecting the better toleration of very high pressures in women, which has long been obvious to all clinicians.

INITIATING AND CONTINUING TREATMENT IN THE ELDERLY

It is important to remember that the clinical problems associated with initiating antihypertensive treatment in the elderly differ from those of continuing treatment originally begun in middle age. As whole populations are more completely screened, decisions to start or withhold treatment in the elderly should become less frequent. Few people develop hypertension as a clinical problem for the first time in old age, and most of those who need treatment should already be having it.

CONTROLLED TRIALS OF TREATMENT INITIATED IN THE ELDERLY

There are now two major randomised controlled trials of antihypertensive treatment initiated in the elderly, the European Working Party on high blood pressure in the elderly (EWPHE) multicentre hospital trial (Amery et al 1985), and John Coope's multicentre trial in general practice (Coope & Warrender 1986). Coope's trial covered 3900 patient-years of treatment in combined treatment and control groups (about the same as the EWPHE trial) at a mean age of 72 and mean blood pressure 198/98 mmHg at entry, giving a 90% power to detect a one-third reduction in strokes and coronary events.

The results of the EWPHE trial are difficult to interpret, because it was based on patients referred to hospitals for all sorts of reasons and slowly recruited over several years. Probably because the patients had been referred to hospitals for symptomatic illness, death rates from all causes were more than twice as high as in the Coope trial — 2.5 times as high for stroke. The EWPHE showed a big reduction in deaths attributed to myocardial infarction in the treated group compared with the controls, but both groups were so sick that this difference might in part have arisen from with-holding diuretics in the controls; that is, lives were not being saved in the treated group, but were being lost in the controls. There was a 32% reduction in deaths from stroke, and no significant change in deaths from all causes.

The Coope trial showed no reduction in deaths from myocardial infarction, but a threefold reduction in fatal strokes and a 42% reduction in all strokes. Episodes of fatal ventricular failure were not significantly changed, and non-fatal episodes were reduced by the surprisingly low figure of 38%. There was no reduction in deaths from all causes.

Two further large randomised controlled trials of antihypertensive treatment in the elderly have yet to be reported — the MRC trial and the systolic hypertension trial in the USA — which will give better evidence on particular subsets. Meanwhile, what practical conclusion can we draw from these two studies, the EWPHE trial and Coope's trial? The absence of any difference in either study in death rates from all causes makes a good case for non-intervention in previously untreated elderly hypertensives without evidence of organ damage. Reduction of coronary risk at this age, even if this is possible (which seems extremely doubtful) seems rather absurd; we all have to die somehow, and this exit seems better than most. A strong family history of stroke should perhaps tip the balance in favour of intervention, but in general it seems to me that the risks both of intervention and non-intervention should be discussed frankly with patients and sometimes with their relatives, who should then make their own choice.

Continuation of antihypertensive treatment already established in middle age is a different matter. This group presumably includes many people who without medication would not have survived, and these trials of hitherto untreated survivors cannot be applied to them.

ANTIHYPERTENSIVE MEDICATION IN THE ELDERLY

Choice of antihypertensive drugs in the elderly should be influenced less by age than by accumulated other pathology. So many old people are already depressed or have diabetes, hyperuricaemia, or severe airways obstruction, that choice is always more limited than in younger patients. Unless there is a strong contraindication, thiazide diuretics are usually a best first choice. If they are not sufficient, beta-blockers are usually well tolerated if reversible airways obstruction has been excluded. Blood levels of beta-blockers are much more variable in the elderly, and titration may be necessary for many weeks to find an optimum dose. Methyldopa is effective in a single evening dose, when its hypnotic effect may be welcome. With a starting dose of 125 mg it is tolerated by about three-quarters of all elderly patients (Ramsay 1981). Postural hypotension is an increased risk in the elderly, particularly in diabetics, and it is probably best to avoid prazosin. Nifedipine is usually well tolerated, and like beta-blockers it is useful for concomitant angina. Reserpine is very effective in combination with thiazides. Active search for depression is essential for all elderly hypertensive patients at every follow-up visit.

IS REDUCTION OF PRESSURE EVER DANGEROUS IN THE ELDERLY?

John Coope's trial (Coope et al 1986), contrary to all expectation, showed no difference in symptoms between treated cases and untreated controls. The authors, rightly sceptical of this result, wondered whether an administered questionnaire on side-effects might be too coarse an instrument to perceive additional symptoms in an age-group in which virtually everyone has aches, pains and weakness, even without medical intervention. However, this result did seem to exclude any very dramatic symptomatic impairments in elderly patients treated with beta-blockers (atenolol) and diuretics, and was supported by the much smaller Australian trial of treatment of mild hypertension in the elderly (Management Committee 1981), which showed no difference in symptoms between treated and placebo groups. One interpretation of both these studies would be that elderly people are helped by regular medical supervision of any kind, even if no drugs are prescribed; or perhaps isolated non-consulters are less active and eat a poorer diet.

However, there is no doubt at all that reduction in arterial pressure can be harmful if it occurs faster than autoregulation of brain perfusion can adapt (Wollner et al 1979), and elderly patients already complaining of transient spells of vertigo and ataxia are particularly likely to be started on antihypertensive medication, though arrhythmias are in fact much more likely causes of these symptoms than high blood pressure, and should be investigated. Many strokes seem to be precipitated by hypotension caused by extracranial events such as heart failure, gastrointestinal haemorrhage, or multiple pulmonary emboli (Mitchinson 1980), and there seems no reason to doubt that incautious prescription of antihypertensive drugs can act in the same way. The answer is always to start with the smallest possible doses of single drugs, with slow incremental titration against blood pressure response at intervals not less than a week. True hypertensive emergencies (in the sense that reduction of pressure is an over-riding priority) are rare at any age, and rarer still in the elderly.

However, the last word certainly has not been said on the potential benefits of antihypertensive treatment in the elderly, particularly when it is begun before the eighth decade. Though a majority of all patients with severe dementia have degenerative disease of the Alzheimer type (Kay et al 1970), most demented men under 75 have multi-infract dimentia (Bergman 1980). Once common in my local population, my subjective impression is that this has almost vanished since we achieved virtually full control of hypertension in the sixth and seventh decades. Evidence of this will be provided by the MRC trial of antihypertensive medication in the elderly, which includes tests of mental function.

WHEN AND HOW TO CONTINUE TREATMENT

Where control of hypertension has been achieved in middle age there is seldom any need for change in treatment through the seventh decade unless onset of angina requires treatment in its own right (usually with a beta-blocker or nifedipine), or blood pressure falls after myocardial infarction. Over the age of 70, however, long-term medication begun in middle age should be systematically reviewed. Around this time there are important physiopathological changes, including a sharp fall in creatinine clearance and slowed hepatic metabolism which can easily result in higher plasma concentrations of many drugs despite unchanged dosage. Adverse drug reactions of all kinds have been shown to occur in about 4–10% of patients at age 25, rising to 7–12% at 60 and 21–24% at 80 (Seidl et al 1966; Hurwitz 1969), and account for about 10% of all admissions to geriatric wards (Williamson & Chapin 1980). As the risks of overdosage and adverse side-effects rise, target resistance falls; control of blood pressure usually becomes easier over time, and excessive reduction occurs more and more easily as elderly patients grow older. Occasionally it may be possible to stop treatment in the seventh decade without return to pretreatment pressures, though in my experience all of these eventually do return to their original pressures within a year. Where a trial of no treatment is undertaken, it is prudent to substitute a placebo during 6 months of regular observation before finally discarding all medication; if treatment has to be resumed, the hard-learned habits of regular medication will then be unimpaired. More often review leads to reduction in dosage, or a change to simpler medication.

A dangerous time for all hypertensives, but particularly for the elderly, is transfer to a new doctor. Confronted by an unknown patient, with a currently normal pressure, before the previous GP's record is available, and perhaps giving an account of previous care suggesting casual supervision, it is easy to assume that treatment is probably not and perhaps never was necessary. All too often this is true, but follow-up a week or two later is not enough to endorse this decision; dangerous levels of pressure may take as long as 3 months to return, particularly after withdrawal of beta-blockers. It is prudent to maintain any treatment that is well established until the original criteria for diagnosis are available with the arrival of the previous GP record. Per contra, if your patient is leaving your practice, a letter giving the original diagnostic criteria and current medication should be given to the patient to hand to the next family doctor.

WHEN AND HOW TO STOP

There are three occasions when treatment in the elderly should stop.

The first is when it should never have been started. Critical evaluation of the criteria on which the original decision appears to have been made often shows no valid indication for treatment, and this is particularly frequent in the elderly.

The second is when treatment is getting too easy. If smaller doses maintain pressure below target levels, they should be reduced further and eventually discarded. A common reason for this is the onset of heart failure.

The third is when treatment is getting too difficult. All the achievements of precise geriatric medicine notwithstanding, people still die of old age, and we are no longer nonsensically discouraged from recording senility as a cause of death. There are few old people on antihypertensive drugs who do not feel a little better without them, and when the game is no longer worth the candle they should be withdrawn.

The most difficult dilemma is presented by brain failure. Where dementia is of gradual and relentless progression, without the relapses and remissions of multiple infarcts, antihypertensive drugs should be stopped. Prolonged survival with Alzheimer's disease is worse than death from stroke, and prolonged survival after stroke with dementia is unusual. Association of hypertension with multiple brain infarcts must be assumed to be causal and therefore worth treating to the bitter end.

REFERENCES

Amery A, Brixho P, Clement D et al 1985 Mortality and morbidity results from the European Working Party on high blood pressure in the elderly trial. Lancet i:1349

Anderson F, Cowan N R 1976 Survival of healthy older people British Journal of Preventive and Social Medicine 30:231

Bergman K 1980 Dementia: epidemiological aspects. In: Barbagallo-Sangiorgi G, Exton-Smith A N (eds) The Ageing Brain. Plenum Press, New York: p 59

Berliner K, Fujry H, Lee D H et al 1961 Blood pressure measurement in obese persons: comparison of intra-arterial and auscultatory measurement. American Journal of Cardiology 8:10

Coope J, Warrender T S 1986 Randomised trial of treatment of hypertension in elderly patients in primary care. British Medical Journal 293:1145

Coope J, Warrender T S, McPherson K 1985 The prognostic significance of blood pressure in an elderly population (abstract). Journal of Hypertension 3:662

Evans J G, Prudham D, Wandless I 1980 Risk factors for stroke in the elderly. In: Exton-Smith A N, Barbagallo-Sangiorio G (eds) The ageing brain. Plenum Press, London, p 113

Haavisto H, Geiger V, Mattila K et al 1984 A health survey of the very aged in Tampere, Finland. Age and Ageing 13:266

Hodkinson H M, Pomerance A 1979 The clinical pathology of heart failure and atrial fibrillation in old age. Postgraduate Medical Journal 55:251

Hurwitz N 1969 Predisposing factors in adverse reactions to drugs. British Medical Journal i:536

Kannel W, Gordon T 1978 Evaluation of cardiovascular risk in the elderly: the Framingham study. Bulletin of the New York Academy of Medicine 54:573

Kay D W K, Bergman K, Foster E M et al 1970 Mental illness and hospital usage in the elderly: a random sample followed up. Compr Psychiat 2:26

Management Committee 1981 Treatment of mild hypertension in the elderly: a study initiated and administered by the National Heart Foundation of Australia. Medical Journal of Australia 68:398

Miall W M, Brennan P J 1981 Hypertension in the elderly: the South Wales study. In: Onesti G, Kim K E (eds) Hypertension in the young and the old. Grune & Stratton, New York, p 277

Mitchinson M J 1980 The hypotensive stroke. Lancet i:244

Ramsay L E 1981 The use of methyldopa in the elderly. Journal of the Royal College of Physicians of London 15:239

Seidl L G, Thornton G F, Smith J W et al 1966 Studies on the epidemiology of adverse drug reactions. Bulletin of Johns Hopkins Hospital 119:299

Spence J D, Sibbald W J, Cape R D 1978 Pseudohypertension in the elderly. Clinical Science and Molecular Medicine 55:399s

Williamson J, Chopin J M 1980 Adverse reactions to prescribed drugs in the elderly: a multicentre investigation. Age and Ageing 9:73

Wollner L, McCarthy S T, Soper N D W et al 1979 Failure of cerebral autoregulation as a cause of brain dysfunction in the elderly. British Medical Journal ii:1117

Appendices

APPENDIX I

EDUCATIONAL LEAFLET FOR PATIENTS

I: What you need to know about your high blood pressure

Your blood pressure (BP) has been found to be high enough to need treatment, probably for the rest of your life. That is a long time. Spend a few minutes reading this leaflet carefully, and then read it again to make quite sure you understand it. Then get your spouse to read it and discuss it together. Next time you see the doctor or nurse, discuss any points which are not clear to you.

Everyone's blood is under pressure, otherwise it would not circulate. If the pressure is too high it damages the walls of your arteries, increasing the risk of coronary heart disease, heart failure, stroke, retinal haemorrhage or detachment, and kidney failure, particularly if you also smoke or have diabetes. *High BP itself is not a disease, but a treatable cause of these serious diseases.*

Unless it has already caused damage, high BP seldom makes you feel unwell. It can be very high without causing headaches, breathlessness, palpitations, faintness, giddiness, or any of the other symptoms traditionally thought to be caused by high BP, and you may have any or all of these symptoms without having high BP.

The only way to tell what your BP is, is to measure it with a BP manometer. This must be done several times to work out a true average, because BP varies so much. If you have a fat upper arm (more than 30 centimetres circumference) BP cannot be measured accurately without an outsize cuff for the manometer; many doctors — both GPs and in hospitals — don't have outsize cuffs, and if they use a standard cuff on a fat arm they may record false high pressures and start you on treatment you don't really need.

Mechanisms

The level of BP depends on how hard your heart pumps blood into your arteries, on the volume of blood in your circulation, and on how tight your arteries are. The smaller arteries are sheathed by a spiral muscle, which makes them wider or narrower according to the needs of the body. In people with high BP something goes wrong with this mechanism, so that the arteries are too tight, and the heart has to beat harder to push blood through them. This tightening-up can occur as a result of nervous or chemical signals, chiefly from the brain, the larger arteries, and the kidneys.

Causes

The causes of transient rises in BP are well understood, but these are not what we mean by high BP. High BP is important only when it is maintained for many years; it is a high average pressure which is important, not occasional peaks. The causes of such long-term rises in pressure are not fully known, though we do know that *high BP runs strongly in families*. This inherited tendency seems to account for about half the difference between individuals.

High BP is also caused by being overweight, particularly in young people. Weight reduction is a sensible first step in treating it. Weight loss depends mainly on eating less fat, meat, sugar and alcohol and more fruit, vegetables, cereal foods and fish. Some of these foods have other good effects as well as helping weight loss. There is good evidence that eating less fat reduces BP, apart from any effect on weight. These changes in diet will also reduce the risk of coronary heart disease by lowering blood cholesterol.

Alcohol (more than eight drinks a day) is a common and important cause of high BP, with its biggest effect in young people. Limiting alcohol to not more than four drinks (glasses of wine, single measures of spirits, or half-pints of beer) a day will often bring high BP back to normal without any other treatment.

Stress

BP rises for a few minutes or hours if you are anxious, angry, have been hurrying, have a full bladder, or if you are cold, so BP measured at such times is not reliable, but none of these things seem to be causes of permanently raised BP. High BP seems to be almost as common in peaceable, even-tempered people without worries as it is in excitable people with a short fuse, but feeling pushed at work or at home may be an important cause in many people, if not for everyone. The word 'hypertension', which in medical jargon has exactly the same meaning as 'high blood pressure', does not mean that feeling tense necessarily raises BP, nor does it mean that everyone with a high BP feels tense. Training in relaxation certainly lowers BP for a while (BP falls profoundly during normal sleep), and probably has a useful long-term effect on high BP in people who learn how to 'switch off' frequently during the day. There is no evidence that treatment by relaxation is an effective or safe alternative to drug treatment in people with severe high BP.

Salt and sodium

Table salt is sodium chloride; it is the sodium which is important for BP. People who eat food with about 20 times less sodium than a normal western diet don't get high BP, and high BP can be controlled by reducing sodium intake to this low level. The diet required for this consists entirely of rice, fruit and vegetables and is intolerable to most people.

The usual British diet contains far more salt than anyone needs, and it certainly does no harm to reduce sodium intake by not adding salt to cooked meals, by reducing or avoiding high-sodium processed foods (sausages, sauces, tinned meats and beans, and canned foods generally), Chinese take-aways (which contain huge quantities of sodium glutamate) and strong cheeses. Milk and bread contain surprisingly large amounts of salt.

There is no convincing evidence that the roughly one-third reduction in sodium intake you can achieve by these changes in diet will reduce moderately raised BP, or that salt restriction of this degree is an effective alternative to drug treatment for severe high BP. However, people with BP high enough to need drugs may manage on a lower dose if they reduce sodium intake, and very heavy salt-eaters should certainly try to cut down. There is much better evidence that reducing fat in your diet reduces BP, as well as reducing blood cholesterol, and you may find it difficult to reduce fat and salt at the same time.

Smoking

Smoking is not a cause of high BP, but if you have high BP already, your risk of a heart attack is increased three times by smoking up to about 50 years of age, and doubled after that age. Heart attacks in people under 45 occur almost entirely in smokers.

Smoking is a very powerful risk factor in its own right, not only for coronary heart disease and stroke, but also for cancer of the lung, bladder, and pancreas, and for chronic obstructive lung disease.

II: When should high blood pressure be treated with drugs?

High BP should be treated with drugs if there is already evidence of damage to the arteries, brain, heart, eyes or kidneys, and in all diabetics. Otherwise it should be treated only if the average BP (calculated from at least three readings on separate days) is at or over about 175/105 (you don't need to know what these figures mean, but you should know what, in your own case, they are, just as you should know your own height and weight). This threshold (or something like it, plus or minus 5 either way) is derived from the evidence of several big scientific trials in Britain, Australia, and the USA, which have shown worthwhile saving of life in many thousands of treated as against untreated cases. Most of the benefit has been in reduced strokes, heart failure, and kidney damage; the effects on coronary heart attacks have been generally unconvincing. The main ways to prevent coronary attacks are not to smoke, and to reduce blood cholesterol.

Drugs for high blood pressure

The aim of all treatment of high BP is not cure (the tendency to high BP lasts all your life) but prevention. People with severe high BP are likely to live longer if their BP is reduced by drugs than if they are left untreated, but they seldom feel better and sometimes feel worse.

People with BP averaging 175/105 or more nearly always need medication to control it, which usually has to be continued for the rest of their lives. All drugs used for high BP cause unpleasant side-effects in some people, though the newer drugs are generally easier to take than the earlier ones. If you think your drugs are upsetting you, say so; there are many alternative treatments. Failure of erection is quite a common side-effect of several drugs in common use, and if this happens make sure you tell the doctor about it; it will clear up soon after your drugs are changed. Other common side-effects are tiredness, depression, and shortness of breath or wheezing. Don't try to alter your medication yourself.

Remembering to take tablets is difficult for many people. Take them at set times, and ask your spouse to help you learn the habit of regular medication. Don't stop them because you're going out for a drink; all the drugs used to control high BP can be taken with a reasonable amount of alcohol. Some drugs used for back and joint pains can interfere with the effect of drugs for BP, and you may need to ask the doctor about these.

Follow-up

Always bring your tablets with you when you see the doctor or nurse for follow-up, so that both of you know exactly which drugs you are talking about. If your BP doesn't fall despite apparently adequate medication, think about your weight or your alcohol intake. Follow-up visits will be frequent at first, perhaps once a week, until your BP is controlled to about 160/90 or less. After that most doctors like to check BP every 3 months or so; never go longer than 6 months without a check.

What about checking your own with an electronic manometer? These machines are easy to use, but they go wrong easily and unpredictably, and unless you know a lot more about high BP than you'll get from this leaflet, you may not realise that you are getting nonsense readings. These machines are useful in helping to decide whether or not to start drug treatment, but don't rely on them for follow-up.

APPENDIX II

Use and care of sphygmomanometers

Blood pressure varies greatly from time to time, depending on the physical and emotional state of the patient. The aim of measurement is to obtain true average resting pressures.

Common causes of *false high* readings are:

1. Anger, fear, pain and embarrassment. The atmosphere should be friendly and unhurried, and with new patients you should explain what you are doing while you do it. Record your impression of the patient's emotional state, if you think this may have affected the reading. Pulse rate can be an indicator of stress and anxiety, and should be recorded at the same time.
2. A full bladder. Ask about this discreetly, if you get an unexpected high reading.

3. Cuffs that don't fit or are badly applied to the arm. The rubber bag inside the cuff must fully encircle the arm. If it doesn't, very high false readings may be obtained. You need at least two sizes of cuff: one for normal arms and one for fat arms. If you are to do your work properly, you must insist that you have these.

Common causes of *false low* readings are:

1. Tightly rolled clothing above the cuff. Many women must take their arm right out of their dress to get a reliable reading.
2. Dropping the mercury column too fast, from bad habits learned in antenatal clinics, to try to save time, or because the control valve on the inflator bulb is leaking and cannot hold the pressure.
3. Pressing too hard with the stethoscope over the artery.

The patient should be sat comfortably with the arm supported on a table. Use *either* the left *or* the right arm on all patients, but not both indiscriminately. Make your readings as accurately as possible. All clinical decisions are based upon them. Lower the mercury slowly, about 2 mm per second (roughly one division on the scale for each pulse beat at a normal heart rate). Write down the pressures as you hear them, or you may find you have forgotten the systolic pressure by the time you reach the diastolic sounds. Make all your readings to the nearest 2 mm down, and avoid reading only to the nearest 0 up or down.

Systolic pressure is the first regular sound your hear. Record it accurately, because it is easier and therefore more accurate than diastolic pressure.

Diastolic pressures is defined either as:

1. the point where the regular, clear, tapping sound is replaced by a muffled, whooshing sound (phase IV),

   or

2. the point where regular sounds disappear (phase V).

Your team must make up its mind which of these definitions it will use, and stick to it. Phase V is easier and probably better.

Patients with atrial fibrillation or very frequent extra (ectopic) beats, will spin off lots of odd sounds above systolic and below diastolic pressure, and BP may be unrecordable. If you notice this, write it down; don't invent a BP that isn't there. In some patients phase IV can't be heard, only phase V. In others the sounds are still audible down to 0. In most of these you can get a diastolic pressure by removing all clothing from the arm, and if that doesn't work, you can try the other arm. If even this fails, if you get the patient back the next day, phase V may be clearly audible. Don't be afraid to record what you actually hear.

How to check and maintain your sphygmomanometer

Errors arise from mercury manometers in three ways: dirty glass tubes, blocked or leaking valves, and leaking tubing and connections. Once every 6 months it should be somebody's job to lift out the glass tube and clean it with the long pipe cleaner originally supplied with the instrument. This will remove dirty mercury from the lumen of the glass tube, so that the mercury level can be read instead of guessed. Next the valve at the base of the rubber bulb should be tested by inflating the cuff and then closing the valve right down. Pressure should hold for 1 minute without much loss; if there is a leak, pressure will fall fairly quickly, and the valve should be opened up and the rubber washer replaced. If the valve seems all right, the leak is probably from a crack in perished rubber tubing, or from one of the male–female joints, any of which can be replaced. When the valve is blocked, usually with fluff, it becomes difficult to squeeze the bulb. The bulb should be removed and the mesh filter cleaned.

APPENDIX III

Protocol for nurse-run blood pressure clinics

(*This is the protocol we have used at Glyncorrwg for many years; it is only a guide, and should be modified to suit your local requirements.*) Blood pressure clinics are held every 2 weeks from 16.15 to 18.00 h. The clinic is run by a practice nurse, with a doctor concurrently available for advice and referral.

Ascertainment, initial diagnostic work-up, and initiation of patient education and treatment are all done in ordinary sessions and should be completed before referral to the blood pressure clinic, which normally deals with people who are already stabilised on treatment and fairly well controlled.

The *aims* of the clinic are:

1. To check blood pressure, medication, body weight, and

current smoking in all treated hypertensives at least once every 3 months.

2. To control pressures below 160/90 mmHg (good control), or 175/100 mmHg (partial control).
3. To verify that patients understand their medication, and if not, to explain it to them; and to enquire about any side-effects suspected by the patient.
4. To control body mass index (metric weight divided by the square of metric height) below 30.0.
5. In patients who still smoke, to enquire about respiratory symptoms, and use these or other opportunities to re-open negotiations on stopping when the time seems right to do this.

Procedures

Whenever a new hypertensive patient is detected in this practice, the patient's record will be marked with a BLUE TAB on the spine, and the name and address will be noted and given to you. Before the next clinic you should enter the name, address, and telephone number, if any, on a card, which you should place in a *boxed card-index* containing all hypertensives known to the practice, grouped in clinic date order so that everyone should be seen not less than once every 3 months. At each clinic each of these cards should be date-stamped, with a note on whether the patient attended or defaulted. No other information should go on this card, except for anything which may help to improve contact. For example, note people who are housebound and will need a visit from the doctor or community nurse, have special difficulties such as odd shifts, or can't sit in the waiting room because of phobic symptoms.

One week *before the clinic*, look through the group listed for it and ask the receptionist to extract these patients' records. Look at the last entry. If the patient has had a blood pressure check within the last 3 months and was well controlled, give him or her a new date 3 months ahead, enter this on the card, and put it back in the box at the appropriate date. If the patient seems to be housebound, ask the practice manager to give the visit either to one of the doctors or to a community nurse, whichever was responsible for the last entry. If the patient defaulted from the last clinic, consider ringing him or her up or visiting the patient at home to find out why it is difficult to attend. For all the others, send out a written invitation to attend the clinic, with an appointment time. Frequent defaulters should be reminded by telephone, if they have one.

At the clinic start seeing patients as soon as they begin to arrive, usually 15 minutes or so before the doctor is due. Enter the date, and if the patient has defaulted or sent an apology, record this. Ask patients how they have been since their last clinic visit, and have a look at the last entry in their record to see if something new has happened since then. Ask the patient to show you his or her anti-hypertensive tablets, which should *always* be brought to the clinic, and check that they are being taken as recorded on the repeat prescription sheet. This is an opportunity to discuss any difficulties they have with the tablets, remembering to take them or possible side-effects.

Then measure and record the following data, both in the patient's record and on the encounter form:

Blood pressure. Use phase V (disappearance of sound) for diastolic pressure, and record to the nearest 2 mmHg, with the mercury descending at a rate of roughly 2 mm per pulse beat. Tell the patient the result.

Pulse rate. Count pulse over 15 s and multiply by 4.

Current smoking in cigarettes per day.

Weight in kilograms.

Peak expiratory flow rate if this was recorded at the last visit.

Ask all patient's if, for *any* reason, they would like to see the doctor. The doctor will be seeing other non-hypertensive patients, but he or she will be under less pressure than you are and *all* patients who want to see the doctor should do so.

Refer patients to the doctor in the following circumstances:

If systolic pressure is over 160 mmHg or diastolic pressure is over 90 mmHg. Before referral, ask the patient why he or she thinks the blood pressure is poorly controlled, e.g. forgetting or lapsing medication, drinking more alcohol, worries at home, and check other medication with indomethacin or other anti-arthritic drugs, or oral contraception.

If pulse rate is less than 60 beats/min.

If you think, and the patient agrees, that it would be useful to tackle smoking again and discussion with the doctor could help in this.

If you think, and the patient agrees, that it would be useful to tackle obesity again and discussion with the doctor could help in this.

If the patient has not seen a doctor for a year or more.

If you are worried for any reason about the patient.

On average, we expect about one-third of the patients to need referral to the doctor.

After the clinic discuss any interesting or difficult cases, and each defaulter, with the doctor. Decide on action to be taken in respect of each defaulter.

Once every 3 months:

Check that every record with a blue tab has a card in the boxed index, and

Check every card in the index to see that everyone in it has either been seen, or that arrangements are in hand for them to be seen.

This will take you an hour or two. If you need more time, raise this at the next practice staff meeting.

APPENDIX IV

FLOW DIAGRAM OF ASCERTAINMENT IN A PRACTICE POPULATION OF 2500

See flow chart page 233.

APPENDIX V

SUGGESTIONS FOR OBJECTIVES AND AUDIT MEASUREMENTS

Experience both in hospitals and primary care shows that rational policies of clinical management (even when fully discussed and agreed by the whole team) make little headway against the inertia of intuitive custom, unless implementation is verified by some sort of audit. This verification should be planned and organised internally, by the same team that elaborated the policies, and is responsible for applying them. Planning, implementation, and verification can and should all be done at the same level of everyday patient contact. Audit is a method of organised, collective, constructive self-criticism.

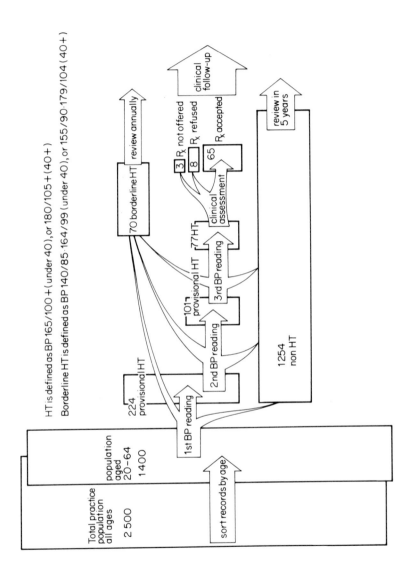

HT is defined as BP 165/100 + (under 40), or 180/105 + (40+)
Borderline HT is defined as BP 140/85 164/99 (under 40), or 155/90 179/104 (40+)

Total practice population all ages 2 500

population aged 20–64 1400

sort records by age

1st BP reading

224 provisional HT

2nd BP reading

101 provisional HT

3rd BP reading

77 HT

clinical assessment

3 Rx not offered

8 Rx refused

65 Rx accepted

clinical follow-up

70 borderline HT   review annually

1254 non HT

review in 5 years

Audit methods of this kind fall conveniently into three groups, all based mainly on analysis of records. All are not essential, and many other methods are possible besides those suggested here. Any would make good trainee projects. The important thing is to obtain valid unbiased data, interpreted by collective discussion.

Random samples of process

These can show how completely the decisions on process have been applied, say 6 months or a year or two after they have been agreed. Examples are:

Of a 10% random sample of records of patients aged 35+:

1. How many have consultations (for anything) recorded during the past year? Of those with no consultations recorded, how many are known still to be within the practice population? Use home visits if no member of the team has any positive information.
2. Of those aged 35–64, how many have arterial pressure recorded
   a. ever?
   b. during the past 5 years?
3. Of systolic and diastolic pressures recorded, how many have terminal digit 0, 5, or other figures?
4. From pressures recorded, construct a histogram to show the distribution of systolic and diastolic pressures at 5 mm intervals, in men and in women, aged 35–64.
5. Of those with any systolic pressure recorded ⩾200 mmHg, how many are in your card-index of treated patients?
6. Of those with any diastolic pressure recorded ⩾105 mmHg, how many are in your card-index of treated patients?
7. Of those not treated, what record is there of the reasons for the decision not to treat?
8. Of the original 10% sample aged 35–64, in how many is information recorded on cigarette smoking? Is it quantified?

Evaluation of process of known hypertensives

Assuming that you have set up a card-index for known hypertensives,

1. What proportion are:
   men under 55
   men 55+
   women under 55
   women 55+

2. How do these proportions compare with the same age categories in your 10% sample? (There are more male than female hypertensives under 55 in the general population. Over the age of 55 there are more hypertensive women than men. Unplanned practice appears always to result in a large excess of women treated compared with men, even under 55.)

3. What proportion of all cases were over the age of 65 when treatment began?

4. How many cases have no record of pretreatment pressure?

5. What is the average number of recorded pretreatment pressures?

6. In how many cases does treatment appear to have been started after only one recorded pressure?

7. Make a list of those under treatment on doubtful original indications, and consider methods of testing validity of treatment in each case.

8. List
    a. the date of the last consultation
    b. the date of the last pressure recorded
    for each patient in the card-index. Analyse these by time-intervals of 3 months.

9. List those who have not been seen for more than 1 year, discuss them, invite them to attend for follow-up, and arrange home visits for the non-respondents.

10. Ask for the reasons for failure of follow up, e.g.
    Felt well and assumed treatment was no longer necessary
    Felt unwell, symptoms attributed to antihypertensive treatment
    Advice from other doctors
    Other advice.

11. In how many treated hypertensives is current treatment recorded? What are your arrangements for repeat prescriptions? Do patients bring their tablets when they consult for follow-up?

12. In how many treated hypertensives have you recorded:
    Pretreatment cigarette smoking?
    Current cigarette smoking?
    Pretreatment weight?
    Current weight.

13. In 30 consecutive patients attending for follow-up of hypertension, treated or untreated, measure pressure with

a standard 22-cm cuff on one arm, and an appropriate (fully encircling) cuff on the other.

Evaluations of outcome

Records of patients who die can and should be retained by the practice for its own research purposes. This is officially permitted, though not widely known. Just let your Family Practitioner Committee know that this is what you intend to do, and do it.

1. Of patients, living or dead, who have had cerebrovascular accidents or transient cerebral ischaemic attacks, myocardial infarction, angina, claudication, heart failure, or retinal haemorrhage or detachment:

   In how many was a preictal pressure recorded?
   How many had preictal systolic pressures ⩾200 mmHg?
   How many of these were treated?
   How many of these were controlled?

   In how many is a postictal pressure recorded?
   How many of these have a postictal pressure recorded ⩾200 mmHg?
   How many of these were treated?
   How many controlled?

   (This analysis assumes a practice disease register. If you don't have one, you can still attempt this by competitive recall using the whole team.)

2. Of your known hypertensives (in the card-index) in how many was the last recorded systolic pressure <160 mmHg?
   diastolic pressure <100 mmHg?

3. Using a self-administered questionnaire, how many of your treated hypertensives

   a. think high levels of blood pressure make you feel bad, and low levels make you feel good?
   b. think high blood pressure is mainly caused by worry and tension, and that if you are not tense or worried, your blood pressure is probably all right?

4. You can also use the self-administered questionnaire on symptoms (Appendix IV) to estimate your iatrogenic cost to your patients.

The results of audit are invariably chastening. Good initial results (more than 50% compliance with agreed policy) are rare.

Good ultimate results, however, can almost be guaranteed, if audit is honestly and imaginatively applied, the results are discussed by the whole team, and initial policies are then modified or reinforced in the light of evidence.

APPENDIX VI

BRAND AND GENERIC NAMES AND UK COSTS OF ANTIHYPERTENSIVE DRUGS

Costs are as quoted in the Monthly Index of Medical Specialties for January 1986. Drugs are listed alphabetically by generic names within groups in the same order as they appear in the British National Formulary. Drugs discussed individually in this book are shown in italics.

Group Generic name	Brand name	Price per 100
Thiazides and related diuretics		
bendrofluazide	Aprinox	0.41
2.5 mg	Berkozide	0.40
	Centyl	1.72
chlorothiazide	Saluric	1.91
500 mg		
chlorthalidone	Hygroton	3.08
50 mg		
cyclopenthiazide	Navidrex	1.77
500 mg		
hydrochlorothiazide	Esidrex	2.50
25 mg	Hydrosaluric	1.46
hydroflumethiazide	Hydrenox	1.75
50 mg		
indapamide	Natrilix	18.75
2.5 mg		
mefruside	Baycaron	15.85
25 mg		
methyclothiazide	Enduron	2.06
5 mg		
metolazone	Metenix	8.75
5 mg		

Group	Generic name	Brand name	Price per 100
	polythiazide 1 mg	Nephril	2.82
	xipamide 20 mg	Diurexan	9.73
Loop diuretics			
	frusemide 40 mg	Aluzine	4.51
		Diuresal	0.50
		Dryptal	1.83
		Frusetic	2.56
		Frusid	1.73
		Lasix	4.66
	bumetanide 1 mg	Burinex	5.43
	ethacrynic acid 50 mg	Edecrin	8.74
	piretanide 6 mg	Arelix	12.03
Aldosterone antagonists			
	spironolactone 25 mg	Aldactone	8.98
		Laractone	4.20
		Spiretic	5.95
		Spiroctan	7.40
		Spirolone	6.27
Compound preparations of potassium-sparing diuretics			
	amiloride/thiazide 2.5 mg/25 mg hydrochlorothiazide	Moduret 25	6.86
	Triamterene/thiazide 50 mg/25 mg hydrochlorothiazide	Dyazide	6.32
	spironolactone/hydro-chlorothiazide 25 mg/25 mg	Aldactide 25	28.96
Beta-adrenoceptor blocking drugs			
	propranolol 80 mg	Angilol	3.81
		Apsolol	0.91
		Bedranol	0.84
		Berkolol	4.16
		$\frac{1}{2}$ Inderal LA	16.00
		Inderal	4.40

Group	Generic name	Brand name	Price per 100
	acebutolol	Sectral	14.56
	200 mg		
	atenolol	Tenormin	24.93
	100 mg		
	labetalol	Trandate	7.94
	100 mg	Labrocol	6.90
	metoprolol	Betaloc	4.71
	50 mg	Lopresor	4.71
	nadolol	Corgard	18.64
	80 mg		
	oxprenolol	Apsolox	5.09
	80 mg	Laracor	5.00
		Trasicor	7.32
	pindolol	Visken	31.97
	15 mg		
	sotalol	Beta-cardone	5.87
	80 mg		
	timolol	Betim	8.77
	10 mg	Blocadren	10.62
Compound beta-blockers with diuretics			
	propranolol +	Inderetic	10.93
	bendrofluazide		
	80 mg 2.5 mg	Inderex	26.57
	160 mg slow-release		
	+ 5 mg		
	metoprolol +	Co-betaloc	23.75
	hydrochlorothiazide	Co-betaloc SA	29.28
	100 mg 12.5 mg		
	200 mg slow- release		
	+ 25 mg		
	metoprolol +	Lopresoretic	12.95
	chlorthalidone		
	100 mg 25 mg		
	nadolol +	Corgaretic 80	31.03
	bendrofluazide		
	40 mg 5 mg		
	acebutolol	Secadrex	26.64
	+hydrochlorothiazide		
	200 mg 12.5 mg		

Group	Generic name	Brand name	Price per 100
	atenolol + chlorthalidone 100 mg 25 mg	Tenoretic	26.57
	atenolol + hydrochlorothiazide + amiloride 50 mg 25 mg	2.5 mg Kalten	23.93
	oxprenolol + cyclopenthiazide 160 mg 0.25 mg	Trasidrex	28.28
	pindolol + clopamide 10 mg 5 mg	Viskaldix	29.18
	sotalol + hydrochlorothiazide 160 mg 25 mg	Sotazide	25.43
	timolol + bendrofluazide 10 mg 2.5 mg	Prestim	13.99
Centrally acting			
	reserpine 0.1 mg	Serpasil	0.47
	reserpine + bendrofluazide 0.15 2.5	Abicol	0.59
	reserpine + hydrochlorothiazide 10 mg	Serpasil-Esidrex	1.88
	methyldopa 250 mg	Aldomet	5.94
		Dopamet	2.67
		Medomet	2.46
	methyldopa + hydrochlorothiazide 250 mg 15 mg	Hydromet	7.60
	clonidine 0.1 mg	Catapres	6.42
Vasodilators			
	hydralazine 25 mg	Apresoline	1.56

Group	Generic name	Brand name	Price per 100
	prazosin 2 mg	Hypovase	6.96
Calcium channel blockers			
	nifedipine 20 mg	Adalat R	19.31
ACE inhibitors			
	captopril	Acepril	23.88
	25 mg	Capoten	23.88
	enalapril 10 mg	Innovace	37.14

APPENDIX VII

DR CHANDRA PATEL'S TREATMENT PLAN FOR RELAXATION TRAINING

The treatment involves training in breathing exercise, deep muscle relaxation and meditation using a biofeedback instrument as a teaching aid, plus educational programmes to motivate patients to practice relaxation–meditation regularly and integrate this behaviour in their everyday life. Instructions for training are on a cassette audiotape. Training can be done by a nurse, and audiotapes are loaned to patients for practice at home.

The educational programme is carried out by the doctor. Patients attend in groups of 8–10 once a week for 8 weeks of 1-hour sessions. The first 15–20 minutes are used for education. The next 30 minutes are used for practising relaxation–meditation. The last 10–15 minutes are used by the nurse to measure blood pressure, and results are fed back to the patient by the doctor to reinforce active participation.

The educational sequence is as follows:

First session: explain treatment plan, the ideas of biofeedback and stress response, and possible subjective, behavioural, and physiological signals which can be measured.

Second session: a film by Walt Disney 'Understanding stresses and strains'. Questions answered. Physiological effects of relaxation explained.

Third session: how and why of meditation explained. Questions answered. Positive effects used to reinforce regular practice.

Fourth session: slides shown demonstrating beneficial effects of relaxation–meditation from other studies. Questions answered.

Fifth session: how to integrate into everyday life. Patients are asked to practise breathing relaxation when stopped at red traffic lights, before answering the telephone, in the dentist's waiting room, or in other familiar stressful situations. A coloured spot is stuck to their wrist watch to remind them to relax whenever they are under time pressure.

Sixth session: protective effects of social support. Cultural and community traditions and communication skills discussed.

Seventh session: type A behaviour discussed. Ciba film 'Stress, personality and cardiovascular disease' shown.

Eighth session: general discussion. Anything patients want to bring up. Regular practice and integration of new behaviours into everyday life re-emphasised.

APPENDIX VIII

HOW HYPERTENSION BECAME A DISEASE

Here are the notes of a medical student, John Spicer, taken at the

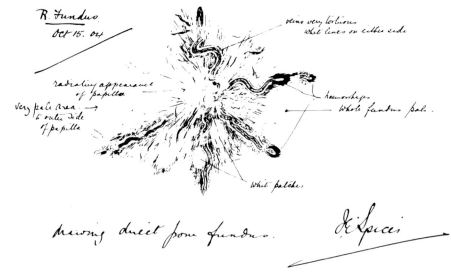

Fig. VIII.1   Extract from the handwritten notes of John Spicer (1904).

London Hospital Medical College, Whitechapel, in 1904. They concern a builder's painter, Thomas Stewart, aged 51 (Fig. VIII. 1).

History

3 weeks ago R eye began to get dim
   8 days ago R eye went quite blind
   Never quite himself since April 15 1903 when he suddenly had a kind of fit while at work. Affected whole R side. Paresis of R side gradually passed off in course of week.

Examination

Decidedly pale, pasty and puffy
   Slight oedema both legs
   Pupils large, R > L
   R fundus shows gross optic neuritis. Very pale retina. Papilla swollen, indistinct outline. Arteries tiny. Veins + + and very tortuous. Neuro-retinitis + +. Much fluffy swelling (oedema). White patches especially to outer side of disc. Many small haemorrhages (L fundus similar).
   Urine: slight amount of albumen
   No intracranial symptoms, headache or vomiting
   Pulse 72, regular. Tension raised, arterial wall thick.

October 17

Seen by Dr Percy Kidd who agreed that patient was suffering from granular kidney

October 26

Patient noted to have blood in R anterior chamber
   Large vitreous haemorrhage with secondary glaucoma
   Pain relieved by eserine

November 2

R eye removed. Very large haemorrhage immediately into orbit.

November 14

No further trouble. Patient discharged.

This case shows the evolution of thought on hypertension. Eight years before these notes were made, Riva-Rocci published the details of the first practical sphygmomanometer. In this teaching hospital everything about malignant hypertension was clearly described except its immediate cause; the pressure itself was not a measured quantity, but a perceived quality of pulse and arterial wall at the wrist. The consequences of hypertension were fairly well understood. They were the disease to which the label 'hypertension' was later appended.

The pioneer in Britain of the idea of hypertension was Sir Clifford Allbutt of Leeds. In his Hunterian Society lecture of 1895 he described, under the now obsolete title 'hyperpiesis', a condition defined by a hard pulse in the absence of renal disease, citing five patients as examples (Allbutt 1896). He had detached the precursor from the outcome, and in the climate of opinion and practice of his day, it inevitably became a disease in its own right. A chapter in the 1909 edition of his own textbook of medicine described:

> Irregular and indefinite perturbations of health occurring in persons on the farther side of middle life, the nature of which is indicated by persistent elevations of arterial pressure. This. . .may persist for years, especially if untreated. . .Sir Clifford Allbutt has watched many individual cases of this kind over many years, years of more or less persistent ailment, insomnia, cerebral confusion, despondency and nervousness, but not necessarily of danger to life. Most of these cases. . .are remediable by deobstruent means. And, although in all the condition tends to recurrence, yet in the less inveterate each recurrence is less obstinate to treatment, and recovery may be anticipated. (Allbutt & Rolleston 1909)

During the first four decades of the 20th century, the sphygmomanometer gradually replaced the finger on the pulse. Sphygmomanometers were still not standard issue to general duty medical officers in the British Army in 1940, on the grounds that though customary in specialist practice, they were unnecessary for GPs; my father's request for one was refused, on those grounds. They were, and to a large extent still are, used not to quantify a graded risk, but to consign consulting patients to one of two groups, those with normal pressures appropriate to their age, and those with a disease, hypertension.

The 'symptoms' of hypertension

By the 1930s hypertension was firmly entrenched as a disease, sometimes symptomless and discovered on routine examination, but often presenting as:

> dyspnoea on exertion, palpitations, a sense of precordial oppression, inability to sleep on the left side, headaches, giddiness, tinnitus aurium, lack of concentration, irritability, anginal pains, epistaxis,

numbness or tingling in the legs, cramp or coldness in the legs . . .
(Beaumont 1935)

This passage is taken from the textbook of medicine which was still used by my predecessor in the Glyncorrwg practice, before I took over in 1961. Hypertension was a handy explanation for symptoms otherwise lacking any negotiable label. The experience of the life insurance companies, and the association with occasional end-stage illness such as that of Thomas Stewart, reinforced the credibility of a diagnosis otherwise as unconvincing as floating kidneys, auto-intoxication from the constipated bowel, visceroptosis, chronic appendicitis, and the rest of the bread and butter mythology of interwar private practice.

Were these the symptoms *of* hypertension, or symptoms *with* hypertension? At diastolic pressures ≥130 mmHg, there is indeed more headache than in controls with average pressures (Al Badran et al 1970). Even then, if pressures are measured routinely in people consulting without symptoms, very high pressures (diastolic ≥160 mmHg) are often completely symptomless. Below diastolic 130 mmHg headache is unrelated to pressure in random samples of the general population (Waters 1971). In hospital outpatients, prevalence of headache has been found to be related to awareness of high pressure, rather than to the level of pressure itself (Stewart 1953).

Robinson (1969) studied the relation of symptoms (headache, dizziness, breathlessness, fatigue, palpitations, insomnia, anxiety and depression) both to the decision of the patient to consult a doctor, and to the decision of the doctor to measure the pressure. The only symptom showing any positive relation to pressure was breathlessness, and this was probably accounted for by associated obesity rather than heart failure. All other symptoms failed to discriminate between 'hypertension' and 'normotension', but apparently acted as cues for measurement, probably because this was the expectation of the patient. Cochrane (1969) studied neuroticism in patients consulting GPs, in relation to the diagnosis of hypertension, and to referral to hospital, using an objective scoring technique. He found that, although there was no association between neuroticism and blood pressure, neuroticism was positively associated with the patient's decision to consult, and even more closely associated with the doctor's decision to refer, regardless of diagnosis. He also found that few patients attending hospital hypertension clinics at that time were referred from GPs; most were cross-referred from other departments.

So here is a 'disease' without symptoms (other than those fortui-tous or prompted by fear) until it has either caused organ damage or is about to do so. If despite this, GPs ascertain it by the selective examination of patients consulting with symptoms traditionally but wrongly attributed to hypertension, the age and sex distribution of the 'disease' as recognised will reflect the distribution of these symptoms, rather than the actual distribution of pressures, and of known reversible risks.

And that is exactly what we find.

Who are treated

Let us look first at the people we do treat. A market research company that has for many years maintained an annual survey of the prescribing activity of an age- and area-stratified sample of 2000 British GPs has shown that in 1968, among those under 65, 49% more women than men were being treated for hypertension, and that half of all those treated were aged 65 or more. The pattern of consultation and prescribing since then is shown in Table VIII.1.

Table VIII.1 General practice consultations for hypertensive disease 1968–1976 (Intercontinental Medical Statistics 1978)

	1968	1969	1970	1971	1972	1973	1974	1975	1976	1977
Estimated total consultations for hypertension, England and Wales (in thousands)	8760	9828	10177	10215	10658	11701	12830	13671	14442	15136
Consultations without any prescription (%)	20	22	20	18	17	18	18	18	19	17
Aged 65a (%)	50	47	58	47	47	47	46	45	44	44
Excess women over men under 65 (%)	49	56	64	60	53	48	53	48	45	44

The pattern is remarkably stable, with only a small shift toward a pattern of diagnosis which is more congruent with the evidence of the distribution of reversible risk in the general population. Over ten years there has been a 73% increase in consultations, and a 63% increase in prescriptions for hypertension, with hardly any change in this irrational distribution by age and sex.

Who are not treated?

The other side of the coin is the evidence on people who are not getting treatment, though on present evidence they certainly need it. Studying random samples of the general population aged 35–64 in South Wales in 1971, Miall and Chinn (1974) found that 18 out of 24 men (75%), and 16 out of 29 women (56%) with diastolic pressures m110 mmHg had never had any treatment, although all of them were registered with GPs under the NHS. Of those who had at some time had treatment, 64% of the men and 32% of the women had begun treatment only after the onset of a major outcome (stroke, myocardial infarction, angina or claudication). Random samples in two towns in Australia in 1971–1972 showed that of people aged 50–59 with diastolic pressures $\geqslant 110$ mmHg only 11% had ever been treated, and 53% had never been told their blood pressure was raised (Lovell & Prineas 1974). In 1963, an authoritative review in the USA estimated that about 50% of hypertension was undetected, 50% of that detected was untreated, and 50% of that treated was not controlled (the 'rule of halves'; Stamler 1973). After a huge and sustained nationwide campaign to change this situation, and a colossal expansion in the antihypertensive industry, studies in Framingham in 1975 still showed that even at systolic pressures over 200 mmHg only 40% of men and 42% of women aged 35–44 had ever been treated (Kannel 1976). In those aged 45–54, only 28% of men and 53% of women had ever been treated, and in the age range 55–64, 37% of men and 40% of women; and all this in what must have been the most heart-conscious area in the whole United States.

In the USA and Australia at least, from the mid 1970s onward there has been a dramatic change in this picture, so that the ascertainment of hypertension in sections of the population with good access to care is far more complete, though there is not yet much published evidence of improvement in sustained control. In Britain there has been steady expansion of both ascertainment and treatment, though far slower and less complete than in the USA or Australia.

Medical trade and medical science

The general picture, then, is one of rapidly expanding activity, in which there is no evidence of any effective strategy to concentrate treatment on those who will benefit most from it, or to avoid interference where it is unsupported by evidence and may well prove harmful. It is still geared to episodic response to symptoms, rather than to needs of health conservation. To change this we must understand why it occurred.

How did it come about that this continuously distributed quantity came to be regarded as a discontinuous quality, a condition that people either had or did not have? How did it come about that a condition that rarely gave rise to symptoms until it had caused disease, became linked in the minds of the public and its doctors with a long list of ill defined feelings traditionally thought to be characteristic of menopausal women, the elderly, and the frightened or depressed of all ages and both sexes?

The reasons lie in the origins of medical trade, and the education built upon it in the late 19th century. The teaching consultants spent their mornings in the great hospitals, giving their services free. In exchange for take-it-or-leave-it treatment of the highest technical quality then available, interesting cases of advanced, end-stage disease, with gross physical signs and every kind of radiological and biochemical disruption, were collected in these museums of living pathology. Here the central features of each disease were defined and taught in their classical form. They were taught as distinct entities, units separate and recognisable in the nosology of disease, as were tigers or cockroaches in the animal kingdom. It was this bestiary of gross end-stage disease that was taught to the students, and which even now forms the core of our beliefs. The 'good' cases were those showing the most florid signs of host destruction, in whom there was least doubt of the presence of an invader. The 'bad' cases (US nomenclature = 'turkeys', UK nomenclature = 'rubbish') were those at the periphery of these central end-stage definitions, at the ambiguous boundary between integrity and invasion, cases that defied simple categorisation. Teaching hospitals were for the poor, who earned their right to be there by their possession of obvious, classifiable, and for the most part incurable disease.

That was in the morning. In the afternoons the leaders of medical thought went to Harley Street to meet their private patients, there to apply to a population with fees in their wallets but less advanced and more ambiguous disease, the simple classification elaborated in the death-house in the morning. These consultants were GPs to the rich. They were involved in a care transaction with a powerful customer in a buyer's market. At a time when doctors could do little to alter the outcomes of illness, a doctor's reputation depended mainly on successful prophecy, and a capacity to both mould and meet the patient's expectations. Central to these skills was application of a label, elastic enough to accommodate a wide range of outcomes, but precise enough to give customers 'scientific' names for their problems, if not solutions to them. The labels used for this generally less advanced, less defined, more ambiguous illness were derived from the end-stage classification of the hospitals. The malignant hypertension of Thomas Stewart, seen in the morning, was the firm anchorage for the unverifiable guesswork of the afternoon. Hypertension was found where it was sought. Doctors believed in what they did; and they transmitted their beliefs to their patients, so that now even we who do not believe conform to the expectations of patients who do. As late as 1973, 36% of a random sample of British GPs still thought that hypertension normally causes symptoms, so that patient demand could therefore be depended upon to initiate diagnosis. There was no significant difference between those who had qualified before 1925, and after 1964 (Hodes et al 1975). The two-thirds who did not believe this still measured more pressures in those complaining of the classical symptoms than those who did not, because they knew that their patients expected them to.

If symptoms do not identify those whose pressures justify treatment, the only rational alternative is that all pressures, in the relevant age-groups, be known. Even this, however, does not of itself evade the consequences of marketed care, as opposed to good husbandry. It is no disadvantage to trade that everyone has a blood pressure; the health-check industry is burgeoning in the United States, without proven net advantage and at the expense of care validated by evidence. Without a fundamental revision of our conceptions of arterial pressure and its control, whole-population screening serves in practice chiefly to lower the threshold of diagnosis and increase the population dependent on doctors. By overloading the medical market with cases of low priority, or who on present evidence do not need drug treatment at all, the number of serious but untreated cases shows little change.

Apparently in all countries (though some more than others) doctors still find it difficult to make quantified responses to quantified risks for disease, rather than the yes or no division appropriate to gross injury. As Sir George Pickering has said, doctors still don't want to count to more than two. If we are to develop the customs needed for effective preventive and anticipatory care, rather than our present ineffective mixture of episodic meddling and heroic salvage, we must discard habits of thought developed to serve an entirely different purpose.

The source of data for natural history is nature, not museums. The enormous debt we owe to our hospitals for the clear definition of disease should not blind us to their shortcomings as a source for ideas about health conservation and maintenance, as opposed to terminal salvage. The complex and usually unknown basis of selection of their cases, their often incomplete follow-up, above all their artificial discontinuity with the population outside, have led to working definitions that cannot be extended to whole populations without modification.

The classical if somewhat vague conception of hypertension as a disease, particularly in Europe, includes progression from a first stage of labile hypertension to a second stage of fixed hypertension. Follow-up of a cohort of 5209 men and women in the Framingham study (Kannel et al 1978), with measurements made twice a year for 20 years, showed that variability of pressure was not a consistent characteristic from one examination to the next (r = 0.07). Variability increased with age, and with height of pressure. To be sure, if we defined 'hypertension' as diastolic $\geqslant 110$ mmHg (or any other arbitrary line), those whose mean pressures are slowly rising will initially fluctuate above and below this line, and later remain above it. In any other sense, the progression from labile to fixed hypertension is a myth, unsupported by evidence.

Slowly at first, but now at gathering speed, the definition of the 'disease' hypertension is becoming an operational one; that is, simply the level of sustained pressure above which we have controlled evidence that reduction is effective in improving net outcome, that health gains exceed iatrogenic losses. The disciplines demanded of treated hypertensives require understanding of the nature of hypertension as a graded risk without symptoms, not a disease. The decision to treat should be the result of measured and matched probabilities of outcome either for treatment, or observation without treatment. Titration of treatment against response should then include the patient's own experience of iatrogenic impairment. Both the decision to treat, and to maintain treatment, should be negotiated contracts in which we are able to give the patient a truthful, albeit simplified, account of probable gains and losses. Science is not about arithmetic certainties, but mathematical probabilities. The latter can be approximated to the former not by strength of belief, but by gathering more and better information from observation and experiment.

Uncomplicated hypertension is not a disease, but its reversible percursor. It is a graded risk factor requiring graded response. How many other 'diseases' will prove to follow this model? And how many other areas in which primary health workers might usefully intervene, have remained at the edge of our attention, because they lacked a disease label?

The figures will compel us.

REFERENCES

Al Badran R H, Weir R J McGuiness J B 1970 Hypertension and headache. Scottish Medical Journal 15:48

Allbutt T C 1896 Senile plethora. Abstract of the Hunterian Society: 77th session, p 38. Reprinted in Ruskin A (ed) Classics in arterial hypertension. Thomas, Springfield, Illinois, 1956

Allbutt T C, Rolleston H D 1909 A system of medicine, vol 6. Macmillan, London

Beaumont G E 1935 Medicine: essentials for practitioners and students. J & A Churchill, London

Cochrane R 1969 Neuroticism and the discovery of high blood pressure. Journal of Psychosomatic Research 13:21

Hodes C, Rogers P A, Everitt M G 1975 High blood pressure: detection and treatment by general practitioners. British Medical Journal 2:674

Kannel W B 1976 The Framingham study. British Medical Journal 4:1255

Kannel W B, Sorlie P, Gordon T 1978 Labile hypertension: a logical fallacy. Abstracts of the 18th annual conference on cardiovascular disease epidemiology 1978. CVD Epidemiology Newsletter 25. American Heart Association, Dallas, Texas

Lovell R R H, Prineas R J 1974 The identification and treatment of hypertensives in two Australian urban communities. International Journal of Epidemiology 3:25

Miall W E, Chinn S 1974 Screening for hypertension: some epidemiological observations. British Medical Journal 3:595

Robinson J O 1969 Symptoms and the discovery of high blood pressure. Journal of Psychosomatic Research 13:157

Bound casenotes of John Spicer, 1904. In the author's possession

Stamler J 1973 High blood pressure in the United States — an overview of the problem and the challenge. In: Report of proceedings of national conference on high blood pressure education, January 1973. Department of Health Education and Welfare 73:486

Stewart I McD G 1953 Headache and hypertension. Lancet i:1261

Waters W E 1971 Headache and blood pressure in the community. British Medical Journal i:142

APPENDIX IX

PROCEDURE FOR CREATININE CLEARANCE TEST

Creatinine is a metabolite of muscle. Daily output and serum levels are fairly constant and to a considerable extent independent of diet.

Creatinine is excreted almost completely by glomerular filtration, hardly at all by tubular secretion, so creatinine clearance approximates closely to glomerular filtration rate (GFR).

Serum creatinine begins to rise above the upper level of normal (110 mmol/l) when GFR is reduced by about 50%.

Creatinine clearance will be calculated by the laboratory from

1. Serum creatinine, estimated from 5 or 10 ml clotted blood, taken at any time, and
2. A 24 h collection of urine. This can be taken conveniently in a 2-l bottle with a funnel, with a few thymol crystals in the bottle to keep the urine sterile. The patient should empty his or her bladder on going to bed (and discard this urine), taking note of the time, and for the next 24 hours all urine must be collected in this bottle. Patients must be warned to pass urine separately before defaecation. At precisely the same time the following night the bladder should be emptied into the bottle and the collection is then complete.

Patients will usually accept responsibility for taking both the blood and the urine sample to the laboratory as soon as possible the next day.

Normal clearance is between 100 and 140 ml/min in an average adult. In children, and at the extremes of height and weight, clearance must be related to these factors, and they should be given on the request form.

APPENDIX X

DETERMINATION OF ACETYLATOR STATUS

(from Schroder H 1972 Determination of Acetylator Status British Medical Journal 3:506)

Give any systemically absorbed sulphonamide in a single dose of about 10 mgxkg body weight. Collect urine for 1 h, between 5 and 6 h later. Send the whole urine collection to the laboratory.

The only problem about this test is getting the sulphonamide, since few wholesalers now stock any of the once commonly used sulphonamides. They all have a long shelf life, so get 100 of any one of them and keep the sulphonamide for the occasional new patient put on hydralazine, after you have verified acetylator status of all your old patients.

APPENDIX XI

A WEIGHT-REDUCING, CHOLESTEROL-LOWERING DIET SHEET

This diet is suitable for people with high blood pressure, diabetes, or high blood cholesterol, and for anyone who wants to reach a healthier weight

There are six golden rules:

Eat less high-energy food
Stop nibbling between meals
Take more exercise
Eat less fat
Eat more vegetables, fruit, and cereals
Measure what you have achieved honestly and regularly

Reduce energy intake

Your body needs fuel to work, as well as other kinds of food for maintenance and repairs. The fuel part of your food we call energy (measured in calories), and that is the sense in which we use the word here. Don't let the advertisers kid you that you need to eat more energy to feel less tired; you would probably feel a lot more energetic if you were eating less energy!

Reducing energy intake means eating less, partly by avoiding between-meal nibbles and snacks, and partly by selectively reducing intake of high-energy foods, particularly sugars (don't forget pop and glucose drinks), fats, and alcohol. Proof that this is actually happening is a slow but steady fall in weight to a target which should be negotiated individually for each patient. Losing a few pounds over the first couple of weeks is usually fairly easy, but the more important aim is a small steady loss of perhaps $\frac{1}{2}$ lb a week over many months, to achieve target weight and stay there. Your new diet is for life, not a gimmick for a quick blitz and then pile it all on again.

Increase energy throughput

Diabetics achieve better control and reduce their coronary risks if they use more energy by taking regular exercise, even if the balance between food input and exercise output remains the same.

Reduce fat intake

Fat (which includes oil, cream, and the concealed fat of cheeses, chocolate, and all fried foods) is not only an extremely concentrated form of energy, but also the main source of blood cholesterol, which is the main cause of atheroma in the coronary arteries, aorta, neck and thigh arteries. Though cholesterol in foods is not good for you, most body cholesterol is made from other fats; what we aim for is not so much a low-cholesterol diet, as a diet that does not generate cholesterol. Some fats raise cholesterol much more than others. In general, fats from farmed animals (saturated fats), both as fat on and in meat, and as milk, cream, butter, hard margarines, and cheese, are all big cholesterol-raisers. Most vegetable fats and fish oils (polyunsaturated fats) tend to lower blood cholesterol. They are contained in corn and sunflower oil, in some soft margarines, and in mackerel, herring, trout and salmon. Processed foods often contain large amounts of fat which are not at all obvious; sausages are often about 50% fat.

There is also good evidence that reducing fat in diet lowers blood pressure.

In most working class diets, the biggest source of fat is frying in general, and chips in particular. The aim should be to reduce fat to about 25% of total energy intake; that is, to reduce the present average intake by about about one-third. You can do this by drinking semi-skimmed milk (which, unlike skimmed milk, you can adapt to very quickly), by eating less and leaner meat, by grilling, steaming, or microwaving rather than frying, and by not automatically spreading butter or margarine on every slice of bread.

Eat more vegetables, fruit and cereals

Plant foods have two big virtues; they don't contain animal fats, so they don't promote blood cholesterol; and they contain large quantities of indigestible residues, commonly called 'fibre'. In fact, as well as fibrous material derived from the cellulose walls of plant cells, they include various indigestible gums which are not fibrous at all, but are equally valuable for a high-residue diet.

The positive effects of these residues are:

to slow down the absorption of food from the gut, so that the pancreas does not have to produce so much insulin quickly; this is important for diabetics.

to make eating harder work; you have to chew more for each

unit of energy taken, so overeating is more difficult.
to improve gut function, preventing constipation and piles, gallstones, diverticulitis, and probably reducing the risk of bowel cancer.

Very large amounts of added fibre, usually bran, can cause quite severe colic and even intestinal obstruction in obsessional dieters who rush into new diets. Plant foods in general, and pulses (beans, peas, and lentils) in particular, produce a lot of gas during fermentation in the gut, and this has to go somewhere. This seems to be less of a problem once your gut gets used to a more vegetarian diet, and the answers are to start slowly, and not to overdo it.

APPENDIX XII

A LOW-SODIUM, LOW-FAT DIET FOR REFRACTORY HIGH BLOOD PRESSURE

When high blood pressure is difficult to control, a big reduction in salt intake will often bring it down. This is especially true of patients treated with ACE inhibitor drugs (captopril and enalapril), which are used only for difficult cases, and may not be effective unless salt intake is restricted. A low-fat diet is essential for all people with high blood pressure, whether easy or difficult to control, because all are otherwise at high risk of premature hardening of the arteries. There is also good evidence that a reduction in dietary fat reduces blood pressure. Low-sodium diets tend to taste rather uninteresting, particularly during the first 2 or 3 months, and unless a conscious effort is made to reduce fat intake, you may find yourself eating a more fatty diet in an attempt to make dull food more tasty.

Salt is composed of two elements, sodium and chlorine. It is the sodium which matters for blood pressure, whether or not it is combined with chlorine as ordinary table salt.

Measuring your sodium intake

Sodium intake is measured in millimoles (mmol). The easiest way to measure daily intake is not to analyse your food, but to measure sodium output, which except in very hot weather is almost entirely in urine, and should be the same as intake. This is done by collecting ALL the urine passed during 7 days, measuring the volume of urine each day in millilitres (ml), and keeping a small sample from each day's collection for laboratory analysis at the end of the week. The exact procedure is given at the end of this leaflet. It looks very complicated at first sight, but compared with the difficulties of reducing sodium intake, it's easy. The results will help you to comply with the diet, and you will find the effort well worth while.

Why do we need to measure sodium intake over 7 days? Why isn't one day enough? The aim is to estimate how much sodium you normally eat and drink on average. Many studies have shown that the amount of sodium people take varies enormously from one day to the next, and measurements based only on one day are likely to be misleading. Average daily intakes in this country are usually around 180 mmol a day to 350 mmol or more; obviously you need to know where you are starting from.

Having measured your intake before starting a low-sodium diet, this procedure should be repeated 3 or 4 months after going on the diet. Only in this way will you know how successful you have been. People who guess how much sodium they are eating are nearly always wrong. In our experience reduction of sodium is difficult for most patients, and you will find it much easier if you have some good evidence that you are achieving something by your efforts.

Achieving your target

If the second measurement shows a daily intake below 100 mmol for an average man, or 80 mmol for an average woman, you are doing all right. How can this be achieved?

Obviously the first thing you will do is to stop adding any salt to your food after it's cooked, and avoid very salty foods like kippers, but salty foods are not the main sources of sodium in most people's diet. Monosodium glutamate is added to many processed foods to improve flavour, bringing Chinese take-away meals to monstrous sodium loads of 200 mmol or more per portion. Generally speaking, off-the-shelf prepared convenience foods tend to contain much more sodium than home-cooked foods. Sodium nitrite is a commonly added preservative, and because the entire food industry is competing for instant flavour-appeal, processed foods are now the main (and not always obvious) source of dietary sodium. For example, one average-sized potato contains 0.2 mmol Na compared with 21 mmol in one cupful of instant mashed potato; one portion of Kentucky Fried Chicken contains 75 mmol, and one portion of branded hamburger and chips contains 97 mmol. Some cough medicines also contain huge amounts of sodium; cough medicines are usually ineffective anyway, the best thing is not to take them. About one-third of dietary sodium usually comes from bread, and one of the first things you will have to do is to find a local source of low-sodium bread or flour. As the sodium content of bread cannot be reduced much below half without making it impossible to bake, even then you will have to limit your bread intake.

Three rules for a low-sodium, low-fat diet

If you follow the following three rules, you should be able to achieve your target. Make your changes slowly, dropping off the forbidden foods one at a time, allowing 3 or 4 months before you reach your target. You will find that gradually your taste changes, so that foods you once thought to be not very salty, now taste too salty.

Stop these very salty or fatty foods, which should be avoided altogether:

Sauces and condiments: Bovril, Marmite, Oxo, chutneys and bottled sauces, laverbread.

Smoked and Tinned Fish: kippers and bucklings, smoked haddock, cockles, mussels, prawns and shrimps, scampi, tinned salmon, sardines and pilchards.

Most breakfast cereals: Weetabix, AllBran, Rice Krispies, cornflakes, Special K, Frosties.

Snacks: salted nuts, pork scratchings, pork pies, pasties.

Most milk products and cheese: evaporated or condensed milk, tinned cream, all hard, soft, or processed cheese other than cottage cheese, salted butter or margarine.

Most soups: canned and packet soups. Though you can cook your own soups with little or no salt, most people find these inedible.

Savoury biscuits and pastry: crispbreads, cheese biscuits, cocktail biscuits self-raising flour, cornflour, baking powder, frozen or packet pastry.

Preserved meats: sausages, fried or boiled bacon, fried or cooked ham, tongue, jellied veal, luncheon meat.

Canned vegetables, baked beans and tomatoes.

Dried fruits.

Golden Syrup, chocolate, toffees.
Ordinary brown, white or wholemeal bread.
Never use sodium bicarbonate when cooking vegetables.

Think about the following salty foods, which you may allow yourself in small amounts:

Porridge, Ready Brek, muesli, Alpen, prunes.
Milk: not more than half a pint a day, yoghourt, ice cream, cream and cottage cheese.
Curries.
Unsalted fish.
Low-salt bread, preferably wholemeal.
Eggs: unsalted eggs don't contain much sodium, but are high in fat and cholesterol. You can allow yourself two a week.
Unsalted butter or Flora and similar polyunsaturated margarines.
Unsalted nuts.

Go ahead and eat as much as you like of the following low-sodium foods. You can liven them up with vinegar, mint and other herbs, spices, mustard, home-made salad dressings, pepper, and lemon juice.

Shredded Wheat, Sugar Puffs.
All fresh fruits, all fresh or home-cooked vegetables,
Rice, fresh meat, fish and poultry, spaghetti and macaroni.

Procedure for making 24-hour urine collections

Each day's collection begins with the SECOND lot of urine passed after waking, and ends with the FIRST lot of urine passed the next day. On DAY 1 the first lot to be passed during the next 24 hours should be passed into the large container provided, which is marked along the side in millilitres (ml). After the first day's collection is complete, read off the total volume of urine in ml and write down the figure. Then pour a little of the urine into one of the small plastic containers. Then pour away the rest of the urine and start the next day's collection, and so on until you have done 7 days, with 7 small containers full of urine and 7 measurements of the total amount of urine in ml. If you keep these in a cool place they can all be sent to the laboratory at once when the collection is finished.

Leave your big container in the toilet you normally use. You will need another smaller container for use when you are away from home, which you can empty into the big container. You will be supplied with some disinfectant, which you should add to each container before you start collecting each day to avoid smells. Be careful with it: it will hurt your skin if it comes into contact.

Remember to empty your bladder first, before you open your bowels. Some people find this easier to remember if they fix a safety pin across their underwear.

You are bound to forget occasionally, and pass some or all of your urine into a toilet. If this happens, estimate the amount you have lost, write it down, and let us know about it when you return your containers to the surgery.

Index